60 tips

cellulite

Florence Rémy

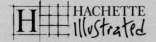

HACHETTE
Illustrated

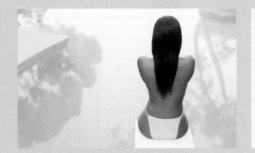
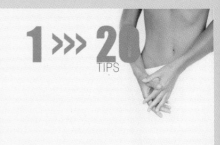

contents

Note: The information and recommendations given in this book are not intended to be a substitute for medical advice. Consult your doctor before acting on any recommendations given in this book. The authors and publisher disclaim any liability, loss, injury or damage incurred as a consequence, directly or indirectly, of the use and application of the contents of this book.

1 >>> 20 TIPS

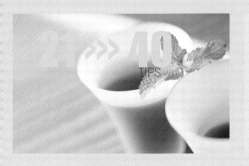
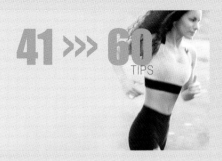

21 >>> 40 TIPS

41 >>> 60 TIPS

introduction

time to take yourself in hand

Cellulite: an inevitable fate?

Whether you know it as 'orange-peel skin' or 'dimpling', cellulite is an unpleasant reality for 95 per cent of women, slim and plump, young and old. Even if you are lucky enough to have beautiful, smooth, taut and flawless skin, one day you may discover the odd lump here and there and realize that the dreaded cellulite is making its first appearance. You will begin to worry about wearing short skirts and trips to the beach or pool.

What is orange-peel skin?

Cellulite is triggered by hormones and is an accumulation of water, fats and toxins just under the skin's surface. Here, adipose tissue (a layer of cells called adipocytes) has a dual function: storage (lipogenesis) and breaking down (lipolysis) of fats.

If the rate at which fat is stored increases, or equally if the breaking down process slows, the adipocytes accumulate fat, then hypertrophy (increase in tissue volume by a factor of up to a hundred) occurs. The fat cells then compress the blood and lymphatic vessels, congesting them and reducing their efficiency. Cellulite can extend over the whole of the lower half of the body, or it may just affect certain areas (especially knees and thighs). Cellulite dimpling appears on the surface of the skin, giving the orange-peel effect.

Multiple causes

A combination of various factors makes a person prone to cellulite.

Gender: first and foremost, where cellulite is concerned, nature dealt you a poor hand if you were born female. Perfectly designed for birth and breast-feeding, even in times of famine, women's bodies are much richer in adipocytes than men's: on average, 23 per cent of female body weight is fat, as opposed to 10–15 per cent in men. Furthermore, women's fat is more commonly distributed on the buttocks, hips, thighs and stomach. Men's is found mainly in the abdomen, and generally appears much later in life.

Genetic heritage: if your mother had cellulite, then the chances are you'll have it as well.

Poor circulation: legs that swell up and marble with veins may be an indication of defective circulation. This favours the appearance of cellulite dimpling (deficient micro-circulation features in many cases of cellulite).

Hormones: oestrogen, especially, and other hormones act directly on fatty tissue. In adolescence, they are secreted in large quantities, promoting the manufacture of fat. During pregnancy and breast-feeding, the fatty tissues change, while during the menopause, the hormonal upheaval favours weight gain.

Repeated dieting: when your weight is stable, you can control the development of cellulite. However, the majority of Western women do not enjoy stable weight. If kilos are shed through dieting but then piled back on once the diet is over (the yo-yo effect) the body is encouraged to store fat in order to guard against what are, in effect, self-induced periods of starvation.

Lack of exercise: hours spent in front of the computer screen, whole days without walking much or breathing fresh air slow down the circulation of blood and lymph, and gradually cellulite sets in.

Stress: it has now been medically proven that stress affects the body's levels of cortisol and catecholamines. Cortisol promotes the breakdown of fat, helps to transport it away from the arms and legs, and reduces fluid retention. Catecholamines (adrenaline) also help in the breakdown of fat.

Smoking: cigarettes aggravate blood-circulation problems caused by the accumulation of cellulite.

Fighting back

Is your cellulite sapping your morale? If it is, do something about it, but don't forget you are dealing with a tenacious problem that won't disappear of its own accord. If you want to gain the upper hand, you must pull out all the stops with a combination of a balanced diet, massage, slimming creams and plants that detoxify and prevent fat storage. Start exercising and tackle the problem right away: invigorated, your muscles will fight back against fat and lost skin tone. However, you must be prepared for a long and laborious battle: you can defeat cellulite, but you will never make it disappear in just a few days with a couple of applications of cream. At the end of your anti-cellulite campaign, however, smooth skin and a slim figure can once again be yours, your posture will be better, and you will be the proud owner of a flat tummy and the lungs of an athlete. Use cellulite as an incentive to adopt a healthier, more active lifestyle while achieving the smooth skin you desire.

how to use this book

This book offers a made-to-measure programme, which will enable you to deal with your own particular problem. It is organized into four sections:

• **A questionnaire** to help you to assess the extent of your problem.
• **The first 20 tips** that will show you how to change your daily life in order to prevent problems and maintain health and fitness.
• **20 slightly more radical tips** that take anti-cellulite measures a little further and help you cope when problems occur.
• **The final 20 tips** which are intended for more serious cases, when preventative measures and attempted solutions have not worked.

At the end of each section someone with the same problem as you shares his or her experiences.

You can go methodically through the book from tip 1 to 60 putting each piece of advice into practice. Alternatively, you can pick out the recommendations which appear to be best suited to your particular case, or those which fit most easily into your daily routine. Or, finally, you can choose to follow the instructions according to whether you wish to prevent problems occurring or cure ones that already exist.

test your cellulite

There are different types of cellulite, including:

- aqueous cellulite (water retention)
- adipose cellulite (often accompanied by excess weight)
- fibrous (or established) cellulite

Find out which type of cellulite you have by ticking **A** if you don't identify with the statement at all or just a little; **B** if you identify with it partially; and **C** if it describes you perfectly.

A	B	C	Slim, but with thick ankles and legs
A	B	C	Plump, with cellulite in the tummy area
A	B	C	Pre-menstrual syndrome makes your lower half swell
A	B	C	Orange-peel knees and thighs
A	B	C	Hips affected, but no pain when pinched
A	B	C	5 kilos (11lbs) overweight, enjoy food, but a bit lazy

A	B	C	Reddish-purple cellulite dimples, painful when pinched
A	B	C	Chunky legs at puberty and after a pregnancy
A	B	C	You play no sport and have flabby thighs that grow bigger each year
A	B	C	Not really fat, but often suffer from bloating
A	B	C	Cellulite that's hard to the touch and some fat

If you scored mostly **A**s, your cellulite falls into the aqueous category: read Tips **1** to **20**.
If you scored mostly **B**s, your cellulite is of the adipose sort: go staight to Tips **21** to **40**.
If you ticked mostly **C**s, your cellulite is fibrous: Tips **41** to **60** should be your first priority.

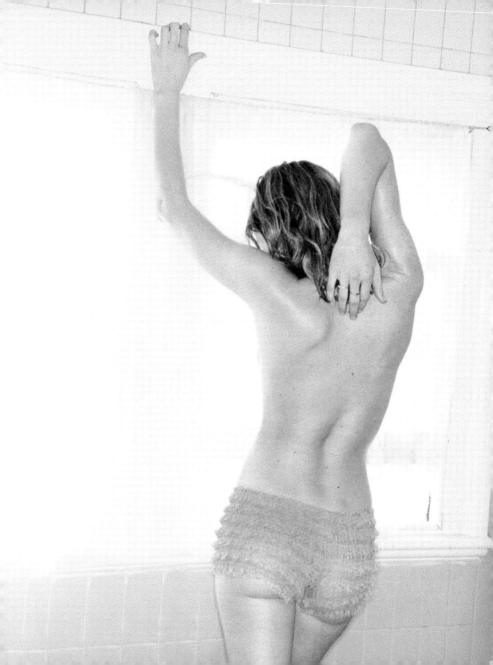

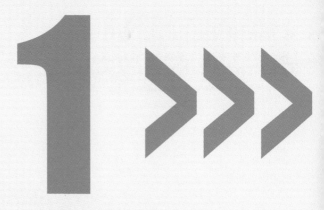

1

》》 You wouldn't admit you had cellulite if anyone asked. But your skin doesn't seem to be as smooth as it used to be. Here and there, you can detect minor changes – your curves and the texture of your skin feel different.

》》》 Define the problem: first of all, weigh yourself. Have you put on a few kilos? It might just be a hormonal imbalance, or a little temporary excess weight, but you should keep an eye on it.

》》》》 You might not have put on weight, but your figure is not what it used to be. Don't let this get you down. 95 per cent of women are affected by cellulite at some time in their lives. But this doesn't mean you have to sit back and accept it. You can combat it.

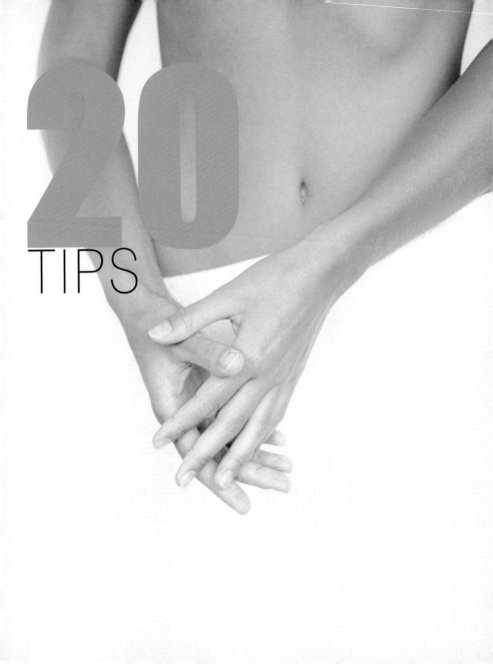

20

TIPS

Describe your cellulite: minor, significant or major. A careful examination will show you the extent of the problem. Be brave and examine yourself intimately, area by area, under a harsh light.

01

identify your cellulite

Close-up

Put one of your legs on the edge of the bath and look at it from the foot to the thighs. Are your ankles a little thick? If you press the skin, do your fingers leave a clearly visible imprint? Can you spot any thread veins along the length of your leg? Are your knees slim or chubby? Standing up, are the insides of your thighs smooth or bumpy? Once you have examined your legs, move on to

● ● ● D I D   Y O U   K N O W ?

> Aqueous (or seeping) cellulite is the most common form. Supple to the touch, it is linked with water retention, oedema of the ankles, heavy legs, varicose veins, poor lymph and blood circulation.

> Adipose cellulite, soft and painless when pinched, appears on the stomach, hips, thighs and inside the knees. It often appears when a few extra kilos have been gained.

your stomach, hips and buttocks. Pinch the skin to find the thickened area (cellulite is sometimes invisible, and the skin only dimples under pressure).

Which stage applies to you?

• **Stage 1** The pinch reveals a little dimpling here and there, but nothing is visible to the naked eye. Waste no time, act fast: you should be able to see results in a few weeks.
• **Stage 2** Lying down, the skin is smooth, but standing up it takes on an irregular appearance, and you have put on weight. Your figure and the appearance of your skin could be much improved with some sustained effort.
• **Stage 3** Standing up and lying down your skin is rippled, and you can scarcely bear to look at the bathroom scales. There's still time to put things right, and there's plenty you can do, but you may need to seek some help along the way.

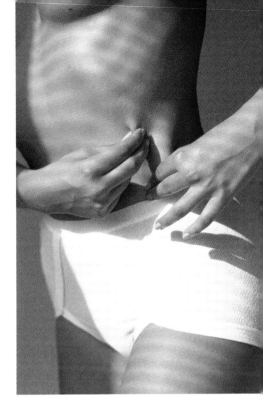

> Established cellulite (dimpling present for over five years) is hard, sensitive and downright painful when pinched. It is prominent on the thighs and knees. The cutaneous fibres (elastin and collagen) are affected.

KEY FACTS

* Don't panic, take a look at yourself and try to pinpoint which stage your cellulite has reached.

* The opinion of a well-chosen dermatologist, doctor or plastic surgeon may be useful.

02

talk to your mother

You might have her smile, her charm and some of her talents, but you might also have inherited much of her body chemistry. 'Look at the mother to learn about the daughter,' as they say. Cellulite can be an unwelcome legacy.

Genetic factors

It has taken years for the importance of hereditary factors to be recognized. Nowadays, with our ailments identified and recorded, our grandchildren will know the family illnesses that may await them, and even at what time in their lives they might strike. Our own grandparents' physical condition might not have been so well catalogued, but family photos are enlightening. See if you can

● ● ● DID YOU KNOW?

> Genetics is the study of hereditary elements and of the mechanism of their transmission. Blue eyes, brown eyes, the shape of the nose – much of our physical appearance and the way we develop is down to genetics.

> Don't confuse cellulite and fatty tissue: the term cellulite describes an increase in the thickness of the subcutaneous tissues. It is possible to inherit a tendency towards plumpness, but not to suffer from cellulite.

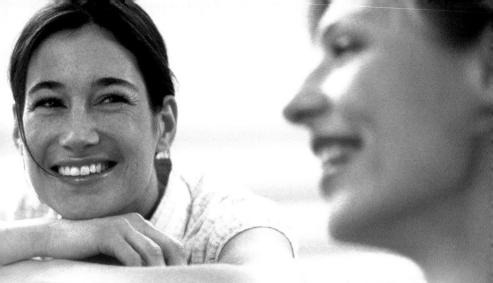

find photos of your grandmother on her summer holidays, in a bathing suit at the beach. It may seem as though you are looking into a mirror, because genetic factors play a highly significant role in the onset of cellulite, as they do in your propensity to put on weight.

How healthy were your ancestors

'Cellulite is often linked to circulatory and/or hormonal problems, so at the first interview I find it useful to ask my patients about their family history', explains dermatologist Catherine Laverdet. Everyone can do a little personal research before a consultation. When asked, your mother will perhaps remember that she had thicker ankles after puberty, that her grandmother had

varicose veins and so on. Quiz her some more and you might learn that, for example, artichokes have always made her retain water, while dandelions seem to help her lose weight. There's a good chance that your body will react in exactly the same way to both plants.

03

From puberty to the menopause, women's lives are influenced by their sex hormones. Oestrogen plays a role in the formation of cellulite. Can anything be done to minimise its effect?

listen to your hormones

A female preserve

Fatty cells (adipocytes) are equipped with receptors that are governed by hormones. 'We know', says gynaecologist Dr M. Lachowsky, 'that endogenous oestrogens [produced naturally by the body], like those of the pill [exogenous], favour the formation of cellulite "balls". At the different stages of female hormonal activity [including pre-menstrual syndrome], water retention can cause the

● ● ● D I D   Y O U   K N O W ?

> Our fat cells (adipocytes) are equipped with receptors that respond to our hormones. These require monitoring during puberty and pregnancy as oestrogen peaks trigger swelling.

During the menopause, the base metabolism is reduced. Without regular physical exercise, energy expenditure decreases and the body tends to grow heavier.

tissues to swell, favouring or aggravating the appearance of cellulite dimpling.'

The pill, pregnancy and the menopause

An unwise choice of contraceptive pill can also lead to cellulite. But nowadays, with the advent of the micro-dose pill, cellulite is rarely a side-effect. One of the latest pills even combats water retention. However, regular visits to the doctor are important if you are on the pill.

Pregnancy often triggers cellulite; and after the birth, the body retains the adipocytes stored during pregnancy. This can be overcome with regular physical exercise, relaxation and a careful diet. During the menopause, HRT (hormone replacement therapy) can have a negative impact on your figure (the heavy legs effect), but weight gain can be restricted if the correct dosage is prescribed.

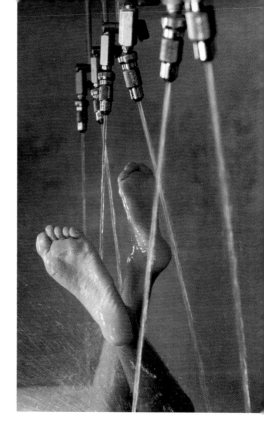

Women on HRT may put on a little weight, but without treatment the weight gain could be even greater, and it might follow the male pattern by being most pronounced on the stomach. There is also an increased cardiovascular risk.

KEY FACTS

* Cellulite that occurs in puberty or pregnancy is the easiest to treat.

* In the case of weight gain or bloating, consult your gynaecologist.

04

say 'no' to crash diets

Not matter how slim you are, if you discover cellulite on your thighs, the temptation is to embark on a starvation diet immediately. But it is now known that excessive dieting is no deterrent whatsoever to cellulite, and may even give it a boost.

Timing and moderation

One recent poll (Ifop, September 2001) suggested that 96 per cent of women want to lose weight. Confronted daily with waif-like mannequins in the media, we are ready to try anything to regain our slender figures. But these days, crash diets are unanimously denounced by experts as inefficient, not to mention dangerous. And in exactly the same way as when quitting smoking, to lose weight you need to choose your moment carefully. Body and mind are inextricably linked. 'Never forget the extent to which emotions play a role in the equation,' says M. Freud, a psychotherapist. If you are eating in response to a specific stressful situation, you should question whether this is the right time to ration yourself.

Proteins and discipline

We generally eat less now than we did twenty years ago but we still do not take enough exercise and our diets are richer in fats and refined sugar. If we want to loosen the grip of cellulite, returning to a balanced diet and taking physical exercise makes more sense than resorting to brutal self-starvation. The only sensible way to lose weight is by increasing energy expenditure through a sporting activity while eating a protein-rich diet (meat, fish, eggs) and keeping your fat intake low.

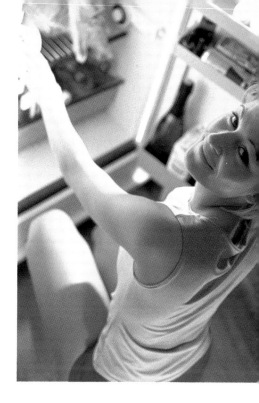

> Before deciding to go ahead with liposuction, some plastic surgeons advise their patients to go on a weight-reducing diet.

KEY FACTS

* Changing your diet doesn't mean starving yourself. To lose weight, you just need to eat a little less of everything.

* Combining a sporting activity with a protein-rich diet is the golden rule for combating that cellulite.

05

evaluate your stress levels

It is thought that stress may contribute to cellulite. When you are tense, your body produces cortisol, a substance that promotes water retention. And even if you eat better and less, stress may well hinder weight loss.

Research the cause

Normally, we adapt to stress, but sometimes it can simply overwhelm us. It's a malaise of the society in which we live, with demands on women's time and attention coming from children, partners, workmates and a host of other sources. The tension mounts, your enjoyment of life fades, your relationships suffer. Measure the stress that affects or devours you and ask yourself a pertinent question: Is the stress the

● ● ● DID YOU KNOW?

> Mental fatigue, anxiety and depression can all cause problems in neuro-endocrinal regulation, which is particularly linked to the formation of cellulite. Stress hormones (catecholamins) push us to increase our sugar consumption while reducing insulin activity.

> Stress leads to micro-inflammation of the blood vessels and promotes the secretion of an anti-diuretic hormone: the body's capacity to excrete toxins is therefore affected.

result of too fast a pace or a specific concern? In the case of the former, you must reorganize your life as a matter of urgency, and give yourself some time to stand back and reflect.

Anti-stress test

❶ When you wake up, are you full of energy?

Yes/No

❷ Do you face your problems calmly and objectively?

Yes/No

❸ Do you have a hobby? (shopping doesn't count!)

Yes/No

❹ Do you refuse to let yourself get upset over small matters?

Yes/No

❺ Do you shut the door behind you without tidying up when you go out to the cinema?

Yes/No

❻ In the evening, do you manage to forget about the problems of the day?

Yes/No

Results:

• If you answered YES six times, well done.
• If you answered YES four times, OK.
• If you answered YES fewer than three times, take a deep breath and try not to crack up.

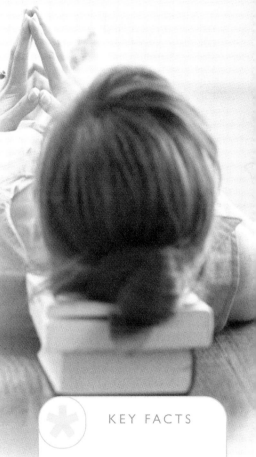

KEY FACTS

* Feelings of intense fatigue, irritability and even aggression are all signs of stress.

* If you are suffering from stress now is the time to take a good look at your life and try to address the problem.

06

learn to relax

Relaxation improves blood circulation, which is very important in combating cellulite. Learn to relax and calm yourself. There are many relaxation techniques; try them and see which one works best for you.

First of all, breathe deeply

A deep breath has an immediately relaxing effect. Tension melts away, the nape of your neck relaxes. It's a habit that everyone should acquire: before you get up and when you go to bed, take several slow, deep breaths. Repeat the exercise at set times throughout the day, and whenever you feel anxious or irritable.

Even better than deep breathing is abdominal respiration. Lying down, knees bent, back flat, breathe out slowly, fully, with one hand on your navel; then inhale slowly through your nose while inflating your abdomen. Hold for a second, then exhale again, still through your nose, while relaxing your abdomen. Repeat ten times.

Inside, do 'the cat' – outside, walk

On your knees, toes on the ground, bring your buttocks down towards your heels while stretching your hands as far as possible in front of you. Put your head on the ground. Hold the position for a few moments, breathing quietly. Take care to align your back and arms.

Set aside ten minutes each day for walking, in addition to a swim and/or one gentle session at the gym per week.

Of all the relaxation techniques that are available, the best is yoga, which is unparalleled. As you have to concentrate on the positions you forget everything else. Also try stretching, and jin shin do (*do-in*), a Japanese self-massage technique that relaxes you and recharges your energy reserves. Contact the useful addresses on page 124 for advice on the best centres in your area.

● ● ● DID YOU KNOW?

> Magnesium has a beneficial effect on your nerves, heart rate, digestive system, immune system, muscular activity and sleep quality. Good sources are winkles, whelks, spinach, artichokes, almonds, hazelnuts, dark chocolate and mineral water.

> B-group vitamins – B1, nick-named the 'morale vitamin', B5, B6 and B9, in capsule form – are vital for managing stress, as is vitamin C, which should be taken in the morning.

> Marjoram, valerian, melissa and passiflora all help too. Take them in infusions or capsules.

KEY FACTS

* Learn to express your emotions: let yourself go!

* Practise a little slow, deep breathing, when you wake up and when you go to bed.

* Reflexology can be a great help (see Tip 45).

07

tone your veins

Malfunctioning veins, so-called venous insufficiency, and cellulite often go hand in hand. Poor circulation in the legs favours the formation of cellulite. Think about going to see a vascular specialist if you are worried about your circulation.

Heavy-legged

Eight out of ten women who see their doctor about circulatory problems receive bad news. 'We examine their legs', explains one vascular specialist, 'and we see varicosity caused by venous insufficiency, together with varying degrees of cellulite.' When the condition cannot be easily diagnosed, a Doppler ultrasound examination is performed to assess the state of the deep veins. Varicose veins are caused by an inherited weakness in the walls of the superficial veins that drain

● ● ● DID YOU KNOW?

> A protein-rich diet strengthens the tissues, particularly the veins.

> Veinotonics, in combination with specific creams or gels, boost the circulation. Red vine (in gel or capsule form) gives relief to heavy legs. Creams containing esculoside (found naturally in horse chestnuts) improve micro-circulation. Buy them at the chemist. An anti-cellulite cream containing *Centella asiatica* combats inflammation.

> Exposure to the sun (heat) and anything that hinders the circulation (crossing your legs, belts, restrictive

blood from the skin and subcutaneous tissues into the deep veins via perforating veins. This can lead to thread veins and swollen, prominent superficial veins, as well as heaviness in the leg and bursting pains after exercise. Modern life and lack of physical exercise exacerbate this problem, which affects many women. If deep veins are involved (usually as the result of a previous thrombosis, often after childbirth) the valves that prevent back flow of blood are damaged, and the result is swollen legs caused by fluid retention and tight, shiny skin.

Walking, a tonic

With many of us leading an increasingly sedentary lifestyle, we clearly do not walk enough. And that's especially harmful as there are major networks of veins in the sole of the foot and the calf. With every step we take, we compress these veins and help the blood return to the

heart. If we don't put in enough steps, this 'return circulation' can malfunction. So, walking has an indisputably revitalizing effect, as do cold showers and kicking vigorously while swimming. Once all that has tired you out, you can also improve venous drainage by putting your feet up.

tights) are not good for your legs. Sitting and standing still for long periods of time without walking also aggravate veinous insufficiency.

> But you do have some allies: anti-cellulite tights and elastic stockings can have a beneficial effect.

KEY FACTS

* A cold shower or a gentle massage helps to keep your blood pumping.

* Walking is the simplest way to achieve good circulation.

08
rethink what's on your plate

Too many women eat on autopilot. A non-existent breakfast, a junk-food lunch, then a calorie-packed evening meal are all too common. But changing your ways is much easier than you might think.

Balance your daily meals

Dietary balance is impossible without respecting the three regular daily meals. **In the morning:** eat a proper breakfast. After eight hours of fasting during sleep, your body needs to recharge its batteries. The good news is that this is the meal that has the least effect on our fat cells. On the menu, include fruit, milk or low-fat yoghurt, wholemeal bread, low-fat butter, cereals, ham (for protein) and light tea.

At midday: don't skip a meal. Have a light lunch, but make sure it is protein-rich, including meat or fish and green vegetables.

In the evening: plan to have a meal that complements your lunch (pasta, for example), and eat fairly early, in a relaxed atmosphere.

Some dinner-party traps to avoid

Calorific bombshells are often to be found on the coffee-table: a peanut contains 50 per cent fat, and ten peanuts equal one tablespoon of oil. Canapes and other snacks, so easy to nibble before the meal, add calories and salt, so reject them in favour of healthy crudités, radishes or cherry tomatoes. When offered a drink, don't be shy: ask for champagne! It's much less calorie-laden

than whisky or a gin and tonic. Remember that many fruit juices are also calorie-laden and are not particularly thirst-quenching. Once seated at the table, even if the food is fabulous, politely refuse a second helping. Use extra virgin olive oil as a condiment as it is high in monounsaturated fatty acids and is thought to help lower cholesterol. Before you crack and attack the cheese board, remind yourself that a splendid dessert might follow. Don't opt for both. Avoid that Irish coffee at the end of the meal, as well.

> Ready meals, fresh or frozen, often contain fatty sauces, and too much salt.
> Choose fillets of fish that you can cook in the microwave with just a little lemon juice.

KEY FACTS

∗ The three meals of the day are important. Never be tempted to skip meals.

∗ Some sugary fruits promote orange-peel skin. Calorie content per 100g (4oz): peach 50; apricot 54; prunes 62; nectarine 64; cherries 68; grapes 73.

09 find the products that suit you

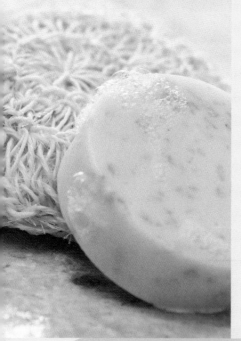

Looking at a pharmacy shelf stacked with tubes and bottles, it's hard to know what to choose. If you have congested tissues due to circulatory problems, the aim is to detoxify and eliminate. Thankfully, there are some very efficient products on the market these days.

> Daily exfoliation is recommended: cleared of dead cells, the skin is more receptive to the active ingredients in the products.
> Pharmacy sales staff should be able to advise you on their products.

Plants from around the world

At the pharmacy, myriad anti-cellulite products offer a profusion of vegetable extracts that claim to be able to decongest the tissues and lighten heavy legs. Some of them (horse chestnut, ivy, holly, horsetail, liquorice and chinchona bark) have enjoyed wide renown throughout history. Others are recent arrivals in the West, such as *Terminalia sericea* from Africa. Essential oils (such as broom and marjoram) are efficient in combating water retention. They can accelerate the circulation, improve the appearance of cellulite dimpling and tone the skin. If you suffer from swollen legs accompanied by fatty cellulite, have a look in your local pharmacy for a product based on geranium (a fat-fighter), Peruvian ivy (which hinders the storage of fats) and liverwort, which boosts circulation.

The wave of marine active ingredients

Other star products come from the sea, and possess natural lipolytic (anti-fat) properties, which can help us to slim. Some product lines available from thalassotherapy centres offer draining baths combining algae (*Laminaria digita*) and essential oils (thyme, rosemary, cypress, lemon). These naturally-based cocktails can accelerate the detoxifying process and reduce oedema. They are also available from mail-order companies in most countries as well as over the internet.

KEY FACTS

* Creams and gels are applied morning and evening (with your legs raised); absorption should be almost instantaneous.

* Some brands can be tried out at spa centres where you can be advised by expert practitioners.

Try to visit them outside peak periods so they've got the time to dispense their wisdom.
> For holidays and weekends away, consider single-application slimming creams.

10 try lymphatic drainage

The lymphatic system is a vital component in the body's waste removal process. Manual or mechanical drainage boosts this function.

'Don't cross your legs!' This advice is often given by doctors. It also helps venous circulation, and is good for the lymphatic system. Unknown by most people, lymph is essential for well-being. It circulates throughout the body, but if this circulation is blocked or decelerated, waste products are not properly eliminated; and veins that are congested with waste products lead to cellulite.

When you rest, put your feet up to help your veins and lymphatic system.

Stimulate your ganglions Physical activity and breathing exercises may boost the lymph, but most effective of all is a specific lymphatic drainage treatment, performed by a physiotherapist trained in the Vodder method, or with the aid of special equipment (some equipment stimulates a reaction similar to natural drainage, acting on the muscles, and is very efficient). Over about ten sessions, the pressure exerted on specific points stimulates lymphatic ganglions, decongesting cellulitic fibres.

● ● ● DID YOU KNOW?

> Lymph provides the cellular system with nutrients and eliminates waste.
> Take care when selecting your practitioner: lymphatic drainage should only be undertaken by skilled professionals.
> Elasticated stockings can perform a similar function on a day-to-day basis.

KEY FACTS

* Make sure that you consult a qualified practitioner.

* Ten sessions should lead to significant results in both slimming and toning.

Pressotherapy is a mechanical massage treatment useful in the treatment of venous insufficiency, oedema and cellulite.

A milder alternative to lymphatic drainage Pressotherapy is identical in principle to manual lymphatic drainage. The results are less impressive, but you will notice an easing of congestion in the affected areas. The technique is performed by a physiotherapist, in beauty salons, at thalassotherapy centres or in thermal spas. The legs are covered by pads wrapped in fabric which are inflated and deflated repeatedly, alternating the pressure and thus boosting blood and lymph circulation.

Relaxing and painless Have one session with a trained practitioner to try out this very relaxing and completely painless technique, but several sessions are necessary to obtain noticeable results. Each session lasts between 30 minutes and an hour, and is followed by a massage. While you are lying down and relaxing, your legs are being toned.

● ● ● DID YOU KNOW?

> This is a passive form of exercise that can achieve firmer, smoother legs and diminish orange-peel skin. The permanence of the results varies, though.

> The procedure is not advised for people suffering from respiratory, venous or heart problems, and high blood pressure in particular.

KEY FACTS

* Don't book a long course of pressotherapy without first consulting your doctor.

* A course of ten sessions will probably be necessary before you see any noticeable results.

It might be quite a while since you last rolled out your gym mat, but get it out again and remind yourself how to loosen up and stretch. Rediscover your flexibility and you will tone up as well.

12

go back
to the gym

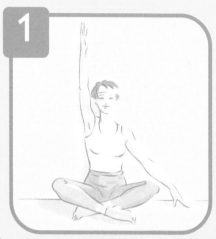

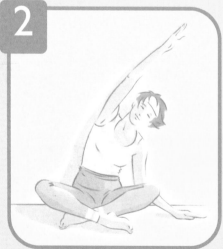

Open up your lungs

① Sit cross-legged, with your back to the wall. Place your hands on the ground either side of your pelvis. Lift your right arm vertically while stretching your chest towards the floor (repeat twice).
② Lean your chest to the left, lift your right arm against the wall and bend your left arm. Hold and breathe. Straighten your chest back to vertical and then bring down your arm (repeat twice).
• Start again, this time with your right arm. During the entire exercise you

should concentrate on breathing deeply. To avoid hyperventilation, always concentrate on a long, slow breath out.

Loosen up your legs

③ Sit down against a wall with your legs stretched in a V shape in front of you. Press down on either side of your right thigh, sliding your hands towards your knee (ten seconds), then from your knee to the start of the calf (ten seconds), then along the length of the tibia towards your ankle (ten seconds).

④ With your arms stretched down your leg, round your back with your head facing your knee. Hold the position for ten seconds. Stand up straight, sliding your hands to the top of your legs.
• Repeat on the left leg, then relax.

Beat stress

Roll a tennis ball under your foot, from the heel to the toes. Start at the outside edge moving the ball towards the inside (2 to 3 minutes each foot). This massage of the sole of your foot is incredibly relaxing.

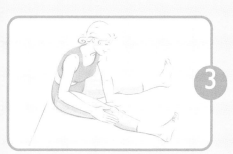 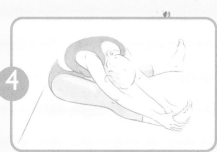

13

flush out those toxins

Drink 1.5 litres (3 pints) of water each day, and, combined with the 1 litre (2 pints) already contained in your food, you can flush out those toxins. Water is a great ally in the battle against cellulite.

Liquid magic

Carrying a bottle of water around in your hand is a good way to remind yourself to drink plenty of water. You should drink 1.5 litres (3 pints) every day. All water helps eliminate toxins, while some mineral waters also contain beneficial elements, such as calcium, potassium and magnesium. Avoid soda water, however, as it is rich in salts that promote water retention.

●●● DID YOU KNOW?

> Every day, the body eliminates around 2.5 litres (4$^1/_2$ pints) of water. All of this must then be replaced. Hydration is vital for the functioning of the kidneys, waste elimination, thermal regulation and the suppleness of the skin. It's pointless to spend a fortune on cosmetic moisturizers if you don't also hydrate your body from the inside.

> Fennel root is thought to sooth the digestion and to have diuretic properties, and recent research has

Tea, herbal infusions and vegetable juices

Hot or iced, green or black, tea is an excellent weapon in the battle against cellulite. Unfermented green tea has stimulant and diuretic properties, as well as a high caffeine content, which accelerates the metabolic rate and contributes to weight loss.

Some plants (whether as infusions or in capsules) are extremely diuretic: thyme, cherry stems, orange-tree leaves, lime blossom, sage, dandelion, briar, meadowsweet. Buy them at the herbalist or the pharmacy.

Cut right down on fruit juices, some of which have a very high sugar content, and avoid nectars altogether. Instead opt for vegetable juices and soups, which are low in calories and rich in fibre and vitamins.

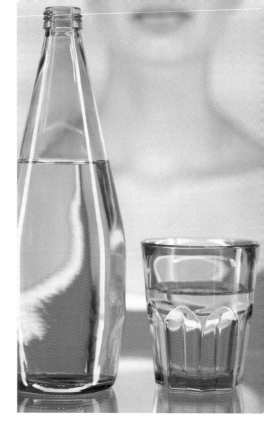

shown that, due to its slight oestrogen content, it might be effective against cellulite and water retention. Furthermore, it does not cause any loss of mineral salts. Buy it at your pharmacy in the form of a fluid extract.

KEY FACTS

* Drink from a bottle. You'll drink larger quantities than if you drink from a glass.

* Drinking water helps you flush out your system and calm your appetite. A good drink of water acts as an appetite suppressant.

14 bin those ashtrays

The professionals are unanimous: doctors and beauticians all agree that smoking aggravates cellulite and wrinkles your skin. It's time to smoke that last cigarette.

The effects of smoking Cellulite is closely linked with vascularization and smoking has a negative effect on microcirculation. Nicotine causes vasoconstriction and reduces oxygenation of the tissues. According to dermatologists, smoking also induces a thickening and drying of the skin, accentuating wrinkles. And, as if that wasn't enough, smokers over fifty are all too likely to see a road map of varicose veins spreading across their legs. The future looks even bleaker when you consider that smokers who take the contraceptive pill are exposed to an increased risk of heart disease.

'But smoking keeps me thin!' No, it doesn't. Look at the statistics. Only one in three reformed smokers gains weight. And even if you are one of the unlucky ones, you'll find that those extra pounds can be shed. More to the point, cellulitic swelling will go down much more quickly. So bin your ashtrays and bank the money you save. You'll soon have enough for a slimming programme and some beauty treatments.

●●● DID YOU KNOW?

> Giving up requires a lot of will-power, so choose the right moment to quit. Get help from your doctor, patches, chewing gum and sticks.
> Smoking affects the body's skin-repair mechanism. For instance, if you have plastic surgery, you are ten times more likely to experience subsequent skin problems if you are a smoker.

 KEY FACTS

∗ New on the market is an anti-smoking stick with essential oils that changes the taste of tobacco.

∗ Consult your doctor, or try an anti-smoking treatment.

15 put your trust in homeopathy

If you are sceptical about homeopathy, feel free to skip this page. If not, read on. There is no miracle homeopathic medicine that will combat cellulite. But homeopathy could still help you.

An environmental issue According to homeopathic doctors, the appearance and development of cellulite denotes a change in the environment of the individual. 'Cellulite develops as a result of a specific reaction to an area of sensitivity, resulting in a need for medicine such as *Natrum muriaticum, Pulsatilla, Kalium carbonicum, Calcarea carbonica* or *Thuya*,' says Dr Jacques Boulet, a homeopath in Paris.

Self-medication Before consulting the doctor, in order to stimulate circulation and the process of elimination, take Fucus and Pilosella (capsules, 2 of each, 3 times a day); Hamamelis composite or Climaxol® (20 drops, 3 times a day); Apis, 15 CH (5g every evening). For cellulite, take Natrum sulfuricum, 9CH (5 granules a day) and 100 drops of Pilosella TM and Fucus TM in a bottle of water, to be drunk during the day (over at least an 8-hour period).

● ● ● DID YOU KNOW?

> Homeopathic treatments can help with anxiety and balance your nerves, which contribute to some forms of cellulite.

> Stress calls for the prescription of supplements or trace elements (manganese-cobalt and lithium), five granules of each every day.

> Several homeopathic laboratories have formulated gels and creams for slimming.

KEY FACTS

* Homeopathy takes a holistic approach to people.

* Before your consultation, make a note of any environmental changes you may have experienced.

16

copy the professionals

Treatments can turn out to be more or less efficient depending on how they are applied. So it's worth spending a few minutes learning how to do them properly.

Prepare your skin

Twice a week, turn your bathroom into a beauty salon. Make sure a chair is close at hand as it is easier to work on some areas of the body in a sitting position. Now all you will need are your beauty products and you are ready to begin. Start by exfoliating using a loofah mitt (thanks to exfoliating soaps, you can now do this in the shower). Once your skin is dry, buff the affected areas (always working upwards), accentuating the movement. Then do a palpate and rolling massage: grip your skin between the thumb and the fingers and roll it. The objective is to increase circulation (the skin reddens). Then, slap your buttocks and thighs vigorously before reverting back to more gentle movements: your skin is now ready to absorb the active ingredients of your treatment product.

Massage and persevere

Apply the cream the same way as the beauticians: put a small amount of the product on the palm of your hand; allow it to warm for a few seconds; then apply it in a circular motion, working from the ankle up towards the hip. For the thighs, think of treating the two sides: first the outside, then the inside (always working in an upwards direction). When you massage your hips, as for the stomach, work in a clockwise direction, concentrating on the parts that protrude most. The active ingredients of decongestants, anti-cellulite creams and toning products will act on your skin.

> Never treat your skin roughly, particularly on your legs. The circulatory system has many little vessels that can bruise or become thread veins.

KEY FACTS

* Preparing your skin enables it to absorb the active ingredients of a cream better.

* Always massage your legs from the ankle upwards.

17

boost your intestinal transit

Half of all women suffer from lazy intestinal transit, and inefficient elimination of waste promotes the appearance of cellulite. But there are several easy steps you can take to address this problem.

Simple measures

We don't move enough, we are stressed and we don't eat enough fibre. (With our slavish devotion to slimming diets, bread has disappeared off most women's menus, which is a shame, because it is a great source of fibre.) The solutions to these problem are obvious, but there are other tactics you can employ, too.

In the morning, when you get out of bed, drink a glass of iced water and then lie

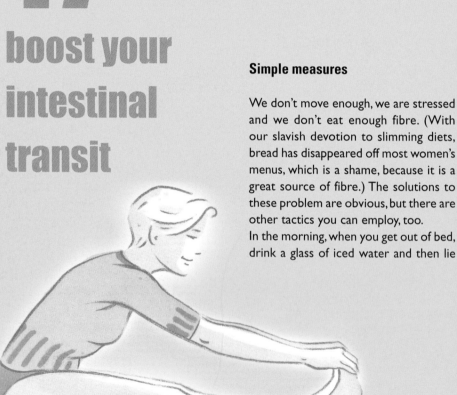

down again for an extra five minutes. When you take a shower, massage you stomach with warm water from the shower head in a clockwise direction. After three hours spent at your desk in the office, get up and go for a walk, breathing deeply and contracting your stomach muscles.

Fast food, literally

You can increase your intake of that all-important fibre by eating soups. Fresh, home-made soup, with chopped vegetables is ideal; make up a large quantity and freeze in small containers. If that sounds like a chore, try frozen or ready-made minestrone instead.

Good transit accelerators are bran loaf, tomatoes, dried flageolet beans, soya, split peas, green beans, leeks, spinach, wholemeal cereals (not sugared), strawberries and raspberries, figs, prunes and fruit compote. Die-hard dieters take note: regularly skipping meals or eating too little will upset your transit, because the bolus (food mass) in your intestines will be too small to be transported.

● ● ● DID YOU KNOW?

> Abdominal yoga flattens the stomach, but it also improves the functioning of the liver and the bladder and facilitates intestinal transit.

> A short exercise: sit down, back straight, arms in the air, legs stretched out, the tips of your toes pointing upwards, without pulling on the thigh muscles. As you breathe out, bend forward and try to touch your toes. If you can't quite make it, it's better to bend your knees a little rather than round your back. Rest for five seconds with your lungs empty and then repeat the position ten times.

KEY FACTS

* Magnesium helps the process. Some mineral waters are rich in this element.

* Among diet products in the shops you will find cubes of fig, tamarind and rhubarb, which all boost transit.

18

free your legs

Inertia, long periods standing or sitting down and heat conspire over the course of the day to make your legs swell. Water retention can be significantly reduced with regular exercise.

Relieve inertia

Standing for long periods is bad for your legs. The return circulation is laboured, as the calf muscle works only when you walk and move your ankle up and down, so venous and lymphatic stasis sets in, the tissue becomes congested and swelling occurs. Relieve oedema by putting your feet up on a chair (but don't cross them) as often as you can during the day. Massage your ankles gently, working upwards. Do some physical activity that

● ● ● DID YOU KNOW?

> Thanks to the pressure of water on our bodies, swimming is top of the list of activities to combat heavy legs. Do the crawl as leg kicking in the water is a great treatment. You don't have to exert yourself too much to achieve a very high level of efficiency.

> When you swim, your body benefits from a hydro-massage which improves your circulation and tones your muscles.

doesn't involve your feet supporting your full weight: cycling activates the circulation, builds muscles in the calves, loosens and slims the knees and shapes the thighs. Three 20-minute sessions per week, alternating a gentle and faster pace, will transform your figure.

Gymnastics, swimming and treatment products

Do some floor exercises. Pedalling is good for the abdominal muscles and the legs; water congesting the tissues passes into the bloodstream and can then be rapidly eliminated. Water massages the legs: in the sea, or the swimming pool, take long steps in water up to your knees; do aqua-aerobics. Afterwards, jog to the pharmacy. Treatments for heavy legs are available in the form of gels, creams and patches. Often plant-based, they boost circulation, providing relief and refreshment. Use morning and evening.

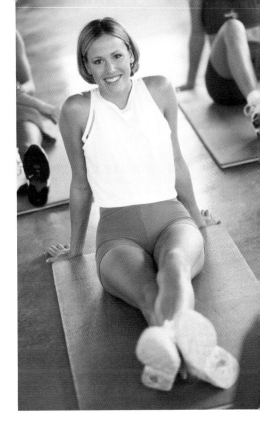

> Smoking and alcohol, spices, too much salt and excess weight aggravate circulatory problems.

 KEY FACTS

* Any physical activity that boosts circulation is excellent, but water-based exercise is best.

* Standing still is detrimental to blood circulation.

* Put your feet up when resting.

19 consume plant extracts

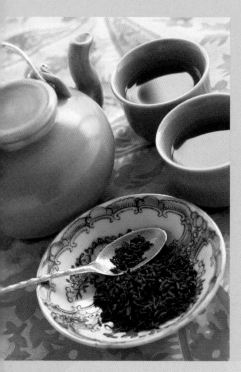

Ancient civilizations were well aware of the therapeutic power of plants. They can form a valuable part of your anti-cellulite programme.

●●● DID YOU KNOW?

> The active ingredients of products for internal use cleanse the body and boost the reduction of excess water in the cells. However, don't use them over a long period of time, as you will risk eliminating essential vitamins and mineral salts as well.

> A reasonable course of treatment lasts three to four weeks, but read the instructions carefully. If you start to feel tired, take vitamin and mineral supplements immediately.

44

Complementary supplements

If you suffer from cellulite and water retention, your objective is to stimulate the elimination of water and toxins from your body. Plants contain many properties that simply cannot be replicated in laboratories, and new ones with a host of benefits are being discovered all the time. They are increasingly present in slimming product formulas in the form of food supplements. For greater efficiency, they often contain combinations of several plants. There are myriad capsules, tonics and infusions on the market. The choice is dazzling, so don't hesitate to seek advice from your pharmacist on the most appropriate one for you.

Top cocktails

The current unrivalled leader is green tea. In capsule form, combined with orthosiphon, it boosts the burning up of fats and combats water retention. Some products combine up to six plants with drainage properties and lactitol, a calorie-free sugar that the body cannot absorb which activates intestinal transit. (Some sugar-free chewing-gums also contain lactitol.) Cider vinegar inhibits the storage of fats. Valuable bouleau marie contains green tea, meadowsweet and apple: it promotes collagen renewal, improving the appearance of orange-peel skin.

Composite infusions should not be forgotten. Some contain algae and plant extracts. They are good starting-points for those with little knowledge of phytotherapy and who don't know which plant to choose. Capsules are often the most practical way to supplement your diet with plant extracts: you can keep them to hand at all times in your bag. But remember to store them in a cool place.

KEY FACTS

∗ Plant extracts, taken in capsule, ampoule and tea form, boost the detoxification process.

∗ Herbal and fruit teas with slimming properties are not by definition disgusting: many have delicious fruity flavours.

> Some specialist treatments comprise both slimming capsules and lipo-reduction gels, with accompanying instructions for how to get the best out of both.

20 chill out

Circulatory activity in the legs can easily grow sluggish. Cold temperatures have a toning effect on the walls of the veins, which contract.

Refresh your legs On a daily basis, end your shower with a series of cold jets, sweeping across each leg, from the ankles up to the top of your thighs. If you have cellulite and water retention, gels or creams formulated to relieve congestion and boost venous circulation (often plant-based), are efficient. Some are even available in the form a patch, to enable them to be applied for a longer period.

Cryotherapy A form of cold therapy that is also offered at some spas and beauty salons, this treatment involves wearing tights impregnated with a glacial gel that immediately reduces the temperature in the legs. It will certainly give you a shock, but it's doing exactly the same thing to any defective, lazy valves in the veins. They are forced to contract and do their job properly. You'll need several sessions before you start to see any results.

● ● ● DID YOU KNOW?

> To be efficient, gels and creams should be applied conscientiously, morning and evening.
> In the evening, sit on your bed with your legs up and apply the product, gently massaging from heel to knee. Wait until it is absorbed, then lie down without putting your feet on the floor.
> Propping your legs up 10cm (4in) in bed at night is good for circulation.

KEY FACTS

∗ Jets of cold water on the legs are very efficient; always work in an upwards direction.

∗ Heated pads and coverings are not recommended.

case study

After going through a bad patch, I felt like I was starting to live again

«Matthew almost made me give up on myself. As soon as he was born, I stopped paying myself any attention, focusing all my energy on him. One day a friend gave me a piece of advice: "If I were you, I'd consult my doctor." I made an appointment. When I arrived, I was in for a surprise: the plaque read, "Plastic surgeon". Was this a joke? I almost went home, but then thought, I've come this far, I might as well see what he has to say. The doctor asked me some questions and examined me. I thought I had put on weight, but he told me it was just slackening of the muscles and cellulite. He encouraged me to do some basic maintenance – diet, more sleep, localised treatments – and advised me to go to a gym twice a week, combining it with aqua-aerobics. I thought I would never be able to do all he suggested, and felt guilty spending so much time on myself, but Neil, my husband, supported me. The result: in three months I've got my figure back (firm tummy, smooth thighs, attractive shoulders), and I feel in top form again. Now Neil has started jogging, too. Matthew is growing up fast. In the end, we're all living better.»

>> **When cellulite is accompanied by excess weight** and the skin is badly affected, localised treatment needs to be more aggressive and accompanied by dietary measures and some serious sport.

>>> Fortunately, **a wide range of solutions are available.** You can dip into them according to your needs, tastes and budget: dietary balance, the gym or adapted exercise, general and localised treatments. The following twenty suggestions cover all aspects.

>>>> **Eliminate more toxins, breathe better, live better**, look after yourself, get motivated to adopt a whole personal rejuvenation programme

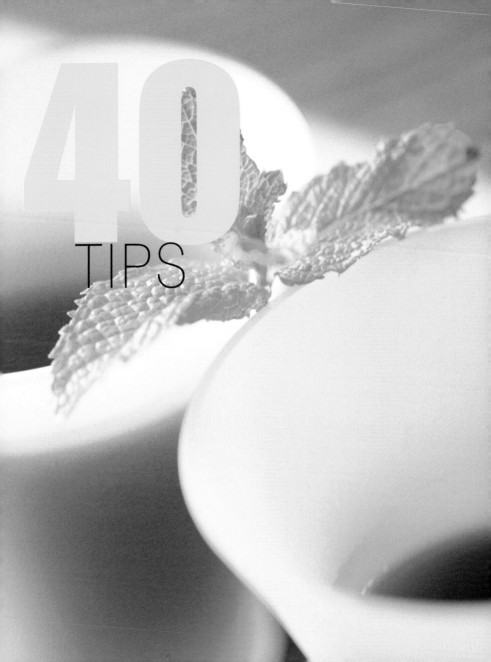

40
TIPS

21

decide to decide

The evidence is obvious. As well as cellulite dimpling, you've put on weight: 3 kilos, 4 kilos, 5 kilos, more? You're determined to lose weight; the decision has been made! Since this is doubtless not the first time, ask yourself why your previous attempts have failed. Which category of slimmer best applies to you?

Six people in search of a slimmer figure

• **The obsessive:** she veers wildly between a normal diet and the pharmacy, feeding herself almost exclusively on tablets, meal substitutes and herbal teas. (That's very dangerous!)
• **The bookworm:** she devours magazine articles and books on the subject, informs everybody of her decision to make her excess weight melt away like

sugar in water. She doesn't think twice about feeding her family nothing but spinach. In short, she goes into slimming mode. (That's not going to work.)

• **The gadfly:** on Monday she spreads herself with slimming creams; on Tuesday she goes on a water diet; on Wednesday she eats nothing but turkey; on Thursday she throws out the salt cellar. (That's not going to work either.)

• **The dreamer:** she convinces herself she can lose weight without changing her diet or cutting out those delicious snacks she loves. (That will fail.) But she decides to go and see a dietician and prove that she has will-power. (That might work.)

• **The activist:** she weighs herself, takes a good look in the mirror, makes an appointment at the doctor's and at the gym. (That might work.)

• **The clear thinker:** she buys a good book on cellulite, reads it from cover to cover and makes a note of what she must do, sets realistic targets and a budget to cover a six-month period. (That *will* work.)

So which type are you?

These generalizations are not as frivolous as they may at first appear. Before your body can change, you might first need to change your way of thinking.

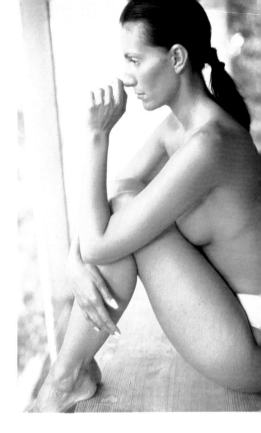

KEY FACTS

∗ You can learn to lose weight in a balanced fashion. A dietary regime can help you.

∗ When you are tired, trying to lose weight is almost certainly doomed to failure.

22

You might think you know your ideal weight, but you could be wrong. In addition to your weight in kilos or pounds, you need to take into account just how much of that weight is fat, muscle or bone. The **BMI** (Body Mass Index) measures body fat in relation to height and weight and helps assess your ideal weight range.

calculate your BMI

Normal BMI or not?

The BMI was introduced by the World Health Organization as a way of measuring excess weight. Your BMI is deemed normal if it is between 20 and 24.9. If it is above 25 but less than 30, you are officially overweight. Between 30 and 35, you are obese. Over 40, you are morbidly obese. You can find your approximate body mass index in the table on the right.

Pounds and ounces
If you would like to assess your BMI in pounds and ounces, there are plenty of web sites that will do this for you. Just type 'BMI' into a search engine and several such sites should be presented.

● ● ● DID YOU KNOW?

> For a precise BMI, divide your weight in kilos by the square of your height in metres, (e.g. if you are 1.65 m tall and weigh 67 kilos, your BMI is: $67 / 1.65^2 = 24.6$ (at the high end of normal). This is only a guideline as the formula does not take into account bone structure or the real weight of your fatty tissue.

Bio-electric impedance is a more precise method, measuring the electrical resistance of the body. Fat is a poor conductor of electricity compared to lean body mass (which has a higher water content), so the more fat, the greater the resistance.

Height in m	BMI = 25 low risk	BMI = 27 increased risk	BMI = 30 high risk
WEIGHT (to the nearest 0.5 kg)			
1.50 (2.25*)	56 kg	60 kg	67 kg
1.55 (2.4)	61 kg	65 kg	72 kg
1.60 (2.56)	64 kg	69 kg	76.5 kg
1.65 (2.72)	68 kg	73.5 kg	81.5 kg
1.70 (2.89)	72 kg	78 kg	86 kg
1.75 (3.06)	76.5 kg	82.5 kg	92 kg
1.80 (3.24)	81 kg	87.5 kg	97 kg
1.85 (3.42)	85.5 kg	92.5 kg	102.5 kg
1.90 (3.61)	90 kg	97.5 kg	108 kg

* height^2: so $1.50^2 = 2.25$

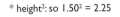

How to use the table

Locate your height in the left-hand column and follow the line to the figure closest to your weight. If you're in the danger zone, consult your doctor; if you're in the increased risk area, speak to a nutritionist.

KEY FACTS

* You are more likely to put on weight from eating badly than eating too much.

* In the case of obesity, hormones, particularly thyroid hormones, might be the cause.

23

consult a dietician

Specialists in the art of eating well, dieticians advise on treatments associated with the diet, often with a view to finding a balanced weight. During the consultation, a dietician will tailor a programme to your needs.

Health professionals

You can be referred to a dietician by your doctor or you may decide to consult one privately, at a health spa or a sports club. Dieticians are expert at devising diets that suit an individual's physical condition, weight and lifestyle, while also taking into account their medical history. They can also prescribe diets designed to treat health issues (diabetes, obesity) or promote weight

● ● ● DID YOU KNOW?

> The first consultation with a dietician starts with a detailed questionnaire on your dietary habits.
> If the desired weight loss is large, medical advice and a check-up are advisable.
> Research a good dietician in your area in the local papers or on the Internet. Your doctor may be able to refer you to your local hospital, especially if you are obese or have other medical problems.
> Slimming clubs may also be of help; group support is excellent for morale and they are not expensive.

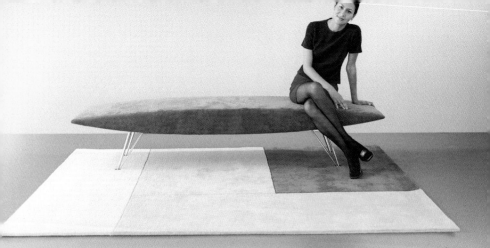

loss. If you want a customized weight-loss programme, a consultation will be worth your while. A specific dietary regime is drawn up after a series of detailed questions have been asked.

Forget your misconceptions

In simple terms, excess weight is stored food energy. If you want to lose weight, you have to address your diet. The target: to establish a balanced diet. It's not so much a case of reducing what you eat, but rather of eating differently, choosing healthy products with a moderate calorie content.

It is a myth that you manufacture body fat only from ingested fat. For example, if sugar is not used up during daily metabolic activity, it is stored as fat. Cakes and pastries contain four times more fat than meat. It's largely irrelevant whether you have steak or chicken for your dinner if you pack your plate with chips every time. But even the meat itself provokes a host of misconceptions: red meat that is not marbled has perhaps 2 per cent fat while that supposedly slimming chicken drumstick has 10 per cent. So you *can* eat red meat: women often lack iron, and slimming relies on a good intake of protein.

KEY FACTS

* The first consultation is aimed at helping you gain an awareness of your dietary habits.

* Dieticians at thermal, marine or health spas have considerable experience in re-establishing dietary balance.

24

lace up your trainers

Cellulite is linked to blood circulation, so anything that boosts the latter is good. And it's impossible to burn fat without proper physical activity.

Endurance sports are a must

Of the average 2,000 calories that we consume every day, 1,200 are used by our base metabolism, 200 are assimilated by the digestion (thermogenesis) and 150 are used for thermal regulation. The remaining 450 are, in principle, burnt during muscular exercise, but, of course, if we don't exercise, we don't need that many calories. Putting on your trainers can't be avoided. Endurance sports are

● ● ● DID YOU KNOW?

> Although an active, sporty person may weigh the same as a plump person, they may look slimmer since activity remodels the figure and muscle is heavier than fat.

> For exercise to be effective and safe, it should be progressive, regular and of a reasonable intensity. Don't push too far too soon.

> Avoid excessive exercise over the summer followed by an abandonment of all sport once it starts to get chilly: by suddenly suspending all physical activity, you will manufacture fat.

> For power walking and jogging, proper trainers are a must.

useful because you don't have to learn a particular skill. You can take up an endurance sport even if you are a bit rusty, as long as you take it slowly to begin with. Cycling, jogging and roller-skating are ideal. Cycling firms and shapes your thighs and buttocks, repairs your veins and reduces cellulite. But if your prime reason for cycling is reducing cellulite, a trip around the block isn't enough. To burn fat reserves, you need to give the muscles oxygen. This reaction is not triggered until you've done approximately twenty minutes of exercise.

One hour, twice a week

All exercise sessions should start and end with some muscle stretching. Then begin your exercise, taking it easy and ensuring you breathe slowly and deeply. Don't worry about taking a break when you feel that you need one. The important thing is to keep it up for long enough: for maximum fat-burning efficiency, exertion should be continuous for 45 minutes (that's when the body starts to dip into its fat reserves). Opt for extended sessions of swimming, cycling or rowing (the latter works 95 per cent of the muscles in your body). Two sessions a week will improve your fitness dramatically, while you slim down.

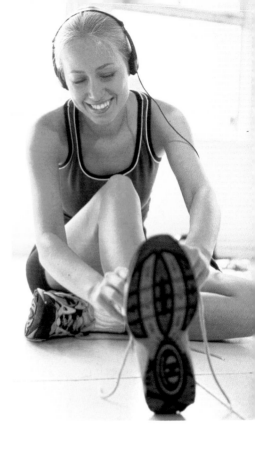

 KEY FACTS

* Exercise combats the muscle loss that results from a sedentary lifestyle.

* Rowing is not recommended if you suffer from back problems.

25 put proteins first

Proteins are essential for the renewal of muscle tissue, bone structure, skin and hair. But do you get enough from your diet, or is there a real need to embark on a course of meal substitutes and food supplements?

If man instinctively became a hunter, it was to meet his protein needs.
> In the long term, following a weight-reducing diet based on proteins alone risks other dietary deficiencies. If you feel tired, stop immediately.

On your plate, at all three meals

Proteins are the mainstay of a sensible diet. You can find them in animal products (meat, fish, eggs), in leguminous vegetables (lentils, peas, beans, soya) and in cereals (rice, wheat and its derivatives). It should form part of all three daily meals. Meat and eggs contain all the amino acids that you need to make proteins. Individual vegetable proteins may be short of some amino acids, and different groups need to be combined to give you the full range of amino acids – cereals and pulses, for example, plus some dairy products. At least one meal a day should contain animal produce (red meat, chicken, fish or eggs), and these foods will keep hunger pangs at bay.

Proteins are invaluable for combating cellulite, as they construct muscle, and toned legs leave no room for cellulite. It is simpler than you think to eat enough protein, but these foods give extra benefits – calcium in milk, iron in red meat, vitamin A and iron in eggs. If you are dieting, choose low-fat dairy products.

> Non-GM vegetable proteins, when carefully used, are a useful and practical way to help control your weight.

Protein in powders, soups or creams

'Pure protein snacks are ideal for many women. Instead of eating an oil-rich Niçoise salad, it's better to open a sachet,' explains Dr Berrebi, a nutritionist. 'But it's important to explain to patients what protein is, the role it plays in muscle development, and in combating hunger, when properly used.' 'Properly used' is the key phrase here. If your objective is to reduce your fat intake, replacing one meal with a protein sachet or soup is a good solution, as long as you also eat a piece of fruit, drink plenty of water and ensure that your other meals are balanced. If you have succumbed to your favourite treat, eating only vegetable proteins for your next meal will help you to stay the course of your diet. Pure protein is efficient in small doses but is not recommended for prolonged periods and you must check the contents of the sachets carefully.

KEY FACTS

* Pure proteins nourish lean mass (muscles) and help you to lose weight quickly.

* Eating proteins (particularly soya) satisfies hunger much faster than eating a low-protein meal.

How do you regain your slim hips and nymph-like, or almost nymph-like, thighs? Some exercises help dislodge cellulite. Here are three of them, to be done three times per week (no less, or you won't see any progress).

26

lift a leg!

Exercise 1

① **Start position:** stand up, legs apart, chest straight, hands on hips.
② Keeping the right leg straight, bend the left leg and drop down as if you were going to sit on your left heel, without arching your back (repeat five times).
③ Start again on the other side.

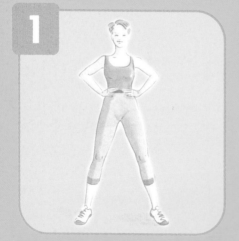

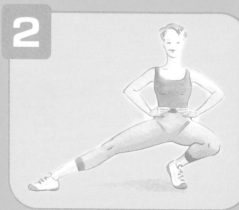

Exercise 2

① **Start position:** stand up, one leg in front of the other.
② Bend the leg in front while breathing out, put your hands on your thighs and come down over your knee while keeping your back leg straight.
③ Wait a few moments. Go back up slowly (repeat five times).
④ Start again, changing legs.

Exercise 3

① **Start position:** sitting down, legs apart, back straight.
② Lift your arms. Breathing in, turn towards your left leg. Breathe out, trying to touch your left foot with your hands.
③ Hold the position for several seconds. Go back to the start position (repeat ten times).
④ Start again with the right leg.

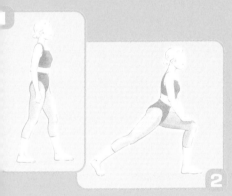

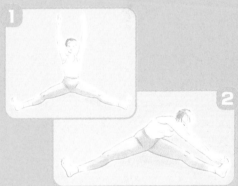

● ● ● D I D   Y O U   K N O W ?

> These gymnastic movements have a relaxing effect.
> Make sure you breathe calmly and follow each session with a short rest.
> Try to do your gymnastics in the open air for added invigoration.

KEY FACTS

∗ Each session should not exceed 15 minutes.

∗ Once you have got the hang of it, put in those 15 minutes every day for the best results.

27

consider acupuncture

Acupuncture is an effective way of combating stress, weight imbalance and the general destabilization of energy. When used in conjunction with other techniques, it can act on cellulite quite efficiently.

An in-depth treatment

Acupuncturists believe our bodies are driven by a vital energy that circulates along meridians. Acupuncture stimulates specific points along these meridians in order to re-establish the energy balance. When treating cellulite, the practitioner must first seek to identify the reason for venous stasis and the stagnation of the fibres and fats (a problem that often dates back to puberty).

● ● ● DID YOU KNOW?

> Acupuncture has been used in China since the dawn of time. Today, it's widely practised in the West, too. Some hospitals offer it as a complementary treatment.

> The needles are inserted in specific points, from the top of the head to the toes, where the yin and yang energies, opposite but complementary forces, circulate, governing the balanced functioning of the body.

A visit to an acupuncturist can be more than just a way of fighting cellulite. It can also be an opportunity to take stock of a situation such as nervousness, poor sleep patterns or weight gain.

Needles, phytotherapy and ultrasound

'With acupuncture,' explains Dr Nicole Maguy, 'you can boost detoxification, improve blood circulation, help with weight loss. In cases where there is a well-established network of fibres, it may not be very effective on cellulite if used on its own. That's why I combine it with other procedures (phytotherapy, trace elements and ultrasound, a very efficient modern technique). In this way, you get really good results in the area concerned, as well as an overall rebalancing of the body.'

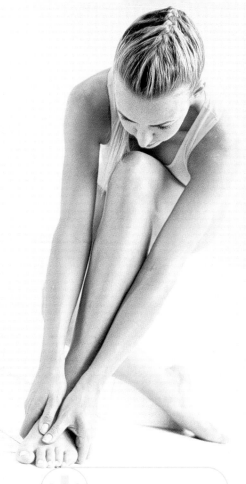

> A word of warning: needles can transmit blood-borne virus infections, such as hepatitis and HIV. Only go to a reputable practitioner who either uses disposable needles or sterilizes them, as is required of any surgical equipment.

KEY FACTS

* Acupuncture is effective against stress, often linked to cellulite.

* This treatment is efficient and safe when practised properly.

28

post-natal cellulite

Carrying a baby for nine months is a wonderful, life-changing adventure, but it has its share of unpleasant surprises. During pregnancy, the body naturally stores fat. After the birth, you may retain a few of those kilos. Many women believe this an inevitable by-product of pregnancy, but it doesn't have to be.

One birth may hide another

Alas, weight gain, a big bottom and the first appearance of cellulite are often the order of the day after childbirth. All of these features are biologically normal, and are part of the body's preparation for breast-feeding – stores are laid down for the baby's future needs. If your body supplies those needs, and you breast-feed rather than bottle-feed, you will lose those gained kilos more easily.

● ● ● DID YOU KNOW?

> You can take a thalassotherapy treatment as early as the third month after the birth, although during the sixth month is more common. Always wait until after the baby is weaned.

> You will receive plenty of advice on dietary balance, relaxation techniques and getting back into shape, as well as information on gynaecological issues. Some thermal spas also offer post-natal treatment.

However, while the fat on the hips and buttocks should disappear, cellulite might be more stubborn. But there is something you can do, if only to put yourself in a better frame of mind to tackle it.

A visit to the seaside

If you are a new mother and you want to treat yourself (after all, you have earned it) try a thalassotherapy treatment. There may be facilities to enable you to take your baby too. Dietary advice is also part of the service, but nothing too harsh, because any deficiency (particularly of iron, magnesium and zinc) must be avoided.

You will be pampered with showers, massages, mud wraps and other seawater-based treatments to tone, oxygenate and revitalize your body and skin. What better way to fight the post-natal blues?

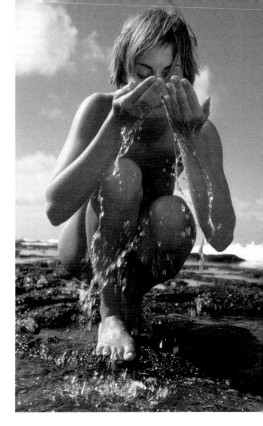

> If you can't go for such a treatment, make enquiries about other treatments such as ultrasound, which gives the best results (see Tip 52).
> In all events, avoid aggressive or deep massage.

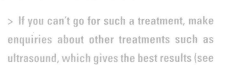

KEY FACTS

* Counter-attack from the first birth; every pregnancy brings its own share of cellulite.

* You will help recover your figure, and feel a newfound energy.

29

go for efficiency

Used on their own, regardless of the promises made, treatment creams can't achieve much. But when combined with a correctly balanced diet and physical activity, they can produce good results.

Targeting specific areas

Gels, creams and lotions are designed to perform multiple functions: accelerate circulation and combat water retention, regulate the activity of fat cells, smooth and firm the skin. Every spring, increasingly efficient formulas appear on the shelves. Retinol-based creams (reputed to have an anti-ageing effect) help prevent wrinkling of the skin. An active biological ingredient, bio-physiotherapy,

●●● DID YOU KNOW?

> The growth hormone that we secrete during the night promotes collagen and protein synthesis (up to eight times higher than that produced during the day).

> Cellulite should recede when attacked by a range of treatments. These products must work in conjunction with a light diet (but not severe dieting, which incites the body to store fat) and sufficient physical activity.

serves as a fat reducer. Molecules from the bark of the apple tree block the entry of fats into the cells, and dissolve those that are already there. Caffeine also works to some extent.

Sleep, and let the creams take care of you

Your body doesn't function in the same way at all times of day. This influences the guidelines for the use of some products which have been developed for use either during the day or at night. A lotion applied in the morning may fight water retention, while a cream applied in the evening can hinder the assimilation of sugars during sleep. Some formulas that combat water retention contain essential oils that also promote the penetration of the active ingredients (to be used in massages).

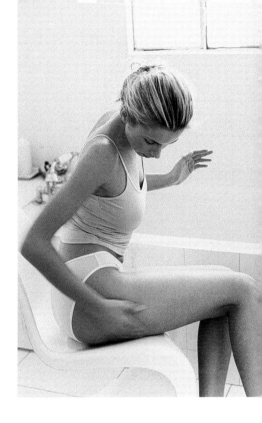

> The massage that precedes and accompanies the application of any product optimizes its effect and, by activating circulation, improves the state of the skin.

KEY FACTS

* Use treatment creams, but don't forget your essential bottle of water.

* Food supplements promoting fat reduction are useful as complementary treatments. See Tip 57.

30 massage devices

Anti-cellulite rollers or massage aids are available from many outlets. They are designed to help expel water and fats from our cells.

Manual massage devices These are available from many outlets in the form of rollers or circular pads. Generally made of plastic or rubber, they have small protusions that massage the skin as the roller passes over it. They are often to be used in conjunction with anti-cellulite cream, massaging 'problem' areas before the cream is applied. In the same way as a normal palpate and rolling massage, they accelerate micro-circulation, enabling the subsequent optimal penetration of the cream's active ingredients.

Electric massagers Motor-driven, these have a handle and big, mobile fingers (with a non-aggressive covering). They massage the epidermis intensively in horizontal and vertical rotating movements, with a deep action. Cellulite dimpling is reduced through drainage, the skin is smoothed, and the whole process relaxes and stimulates. These devices are used on clean, dry skin. Follow the massage with an application of a cream or gel (often supplied).

● ● ● DID YOU KNOW?

> The electrical models act on the legs, thighs, hips and stomach.
> Some creams have knobbles on the caps of their bottles: you massage and apply the cream at the same time. This is especially useful when travelling.

KEY FACTS

* Manual rollers are available at your perfumery, pharmacy or department store.

* Electrical massagers can be purchased at electrical goods stores and by mail order.

31 the truth about caffeine

If you can't get through the day without your caffeine kick, you probably won't be surprised to learn that caffeine possesses other potent properties, too. However, you may not know that one of them is a power to fight cellulite.

Choose green tea Coffee gives everyone a lift, but you will have noticed that the more you drink, the more you need to get the same boost. There is a much healthier alternative source of caffeine. Green tea accelerates urinary excretion, combats constipation and stimulates the mind. You can also drink it safely all day long. Choose one of the organic brands, and, if you can, always make the tea with spring water.

Anoint yourself with caffeine Caffeine is contained in the formulas of numerous treatment products. Of all the lypolitics, it is the only ingredient recognized as being active in lypidic mobilization. Two forms of the substance stimulate lipolysis (reduction of fat storage): base caffeine and caffeine salts. They can be found in slimming gels combined with other active ingredients.

● ● ● DID YOU KNOW?

> Caffeine acts on adipocytes, with its effectiveness depending on the concentration: one of the most effective has a 5 per cent content.

> The latest development in anti-cellulite creams is based on aroma-cology. By smelling these specially fragranced lotions, a message is sent to the brain to produce the hormone noradrenaline. This, combined with caffeine, helps break down fat.

KEY FACTS

∗ Caffeine is credited with the ability to speed up the metabolism and break down fat.

∗ Don't drink caffeine after 4 p.m if you suffer from insomnia.

32 a visit to the beauty parlour

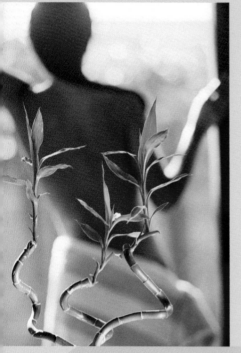

Treatments and massages performed by beauticians are much more efficient than anything you can do yourself on a daily basis. And, of course, everyone loves to be pampered!

● ● ● DID YOU KNOW?

> Many beauticians are trained in techniques such as Thai, Oriental and Californian massage that leave the body in a state of absolute relaxation and ease blocked circulation.

> To aid your relaxation, choose a beauty parlour near your home or workplace so you don't have to rush and battle through traffic to reach it. Some beauty parlours and thermal spas specialize in anti-cellulite treatments. But they all have slimming treatments and products.

Banish stress and banish cellulite

A session at the beauty salon starts with movements intended to relieve tension. Where cellulite is concerned, properly exerted pressure on the stomach and plexus is very useful. In times of stress, the body retains fat and water, and this action relaxes and firms the tissues. Each beauty parlour has its own range of treatments, products and specialities: detox, smoothing, massage, acupressure, relaxation, hydrotherapy, wraps, etc. The products used often owe their properties to phytotherapy, clay, marine extracts and essential oils. A typical session lasts between one and one and a half hours.

Only regular sessions pay off

Don't expect miracles at the first session. Generally, you need around three before you start to notice any effect.

> The most chic and expensive beauty parlours are not necessarily the best. Some highly skilled beauticians work in smaller practices and some cheaper products are very effective without breaking the bank.

Pampering will boost you psychologically, which will in turn have a beneficial effect on you physically. The action on cellulite takes several different forms: treatments and massages are accompanied by mechanical techniques. If you don't fall asleep, talk over your weight and skin problems with the beautician. She will give you informed advice. With regular visits (such as two per week), you might achieve significant results in terms of weight loss and smoother skin. And you will certainly feel lighter and more relaxed.

KEY FACTS

∗ Wear clothes that are easy to remove, and leave your jewellery at home.

∗ An afternoon appointment virtually guarantees a good night's sleep.

33

don't dismiss aesthetic surgery

Sometimes, the best solution is one that many people consider too radical for them. But aesthetic doctors see hundreds of patients each year and they are experienced in some techniques that are very efficient weapons against cellulite.

Adipolysis: salt and ultrasound

After pinpointing the areas affected by cellulite, a hypotonic solution (containing less salt than the physiological serum in which our cells are bathed) is injected. The doctor then exposes the area to ultrasound waves to liquefy the fats, which are subsequently safely absorbed into the bloodstream prior to being excreted. Over fifteen sessions, cellulite

● ● ● DID YOU KNOW?

> These methods represent only a fraction of the treatments available from aesthetic practitioners.
> Although Liposuction is not suitable for all patients, it is an excellent technique to correct normal, but cosmetically unattrac-tive, fat deposits that are resistant to dieting and exercise. Patients should generally be within 10-15% of ideal body weight to achieve maxi-mum benefits, but some patients who are beyond this guideline can also

disappears, blood circulation is stimulated, and the skin is firmed. You should be aware that it can be slightly painful and there may be some bruising at the first session. You will also need two or three maintenance sessions each year.

Liposuction

To remove local fat deposits, small incisions are made in the skin. Saline solution is then injected and may be combined with local anaesthetic to numb the area. After a short time, fat is sucked out through thin needles using a vacuum. (This process may be combined with ultrasound to break up the fatty tissue.) The technique can be performed on an out-patient basis, especially when a local anaesthetic is used, although general anaesthesia might be required. (See also Tip 39.)

benefit. However, Liposuction should never be considered as a weight loss technique. You should try a slimming programme before you consider having liposuction to sculpt your body further.

KEY FACTS

* These techniques are effective on 50 per cent of women and are relatively expensive.

* Whatever the chosen technique, you will always need maintenance sessions.

34

slimming sounds

Music therapy is an alternative treatment that can be used for all ages. A method has been formulated which helps you to slim and stimulates the endocrine glands.

Healing sounds

Certain sounds, voices, tones and music can create a feeling of bliss, while others make us feel ill at ease. Sound therapy is based on the fact that all the cells in our body vibrate at a certain frequency. The cells vibrate at an uneven rate or rhythm when we are unwell. Practitioners believe that by creating soundwaves of the appropriate frequency, the cells can

● ● ● D I D Y O U K N O W ?

> Research at a medical centre for people with Alzheimer's showed that vocal sounds had a significant effect on the patients' endocrine glands.

> It was observed that after four weeks of sound therapy sessions, melatonin levels (melatonin is one of the chemical mediators that determines behaviour) were considerably higher.

be persuaded to regain their correct vibrating frequency. There is little scientific evidence to date to support such a theory, but there is no denying the beneficial effects of music for many people.

Slimming notes

Sound therapy is designed to be used in conjunction with dieting to promote weight loss. Drawing on psycho-sonic techniques, it utilizes the ability of cells, glands and organs to react to sound stimuli. 'Acting on the different metabolic and hormonal functions,' explains the author of a book on the subject, 'the sounds reinforce the efficiency of the diet by improving the assimilation of food.' A CD of soothing, relaxing sounds is played, and the idea is that the listener will no longer focus on their physical state – which is one of hunger – but will be transported to a more spiritual realm.

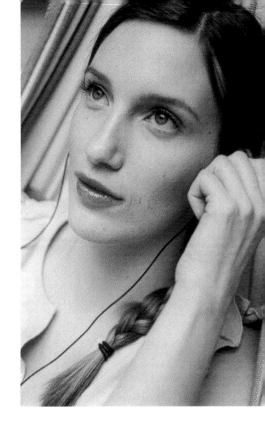

> Music is a powerful tool that can be used in many ways. It has been proven that the type of music that makes a person relax or become receptive is not any one kind. It is dependant on the individual and their own affinity with the music.

KEY FACTS

* Music therapy is an alternative treatment based on the balance between mind and body.

* Each vowel sound corresponds to a different area of the body.

35

dislodge your cellulite

New treatments are being developed all the time, such as body-rolling massage. As with many other treatments, it originated as a medical treatment, but its beneficial effects have now also been adopted in the fight against cellulite.

Non-invasive

This is a non-invasive and non-surgical, motorized, massage treatment for cellulite that is offered by many health spas and beauty salons all over the world. It reproduces the movement of a palpate and rolling massage mechanically, detoxifying and toning the skin, and firming the tissue. It does not remove cellulite, but rather reduces the orange-peel skin appearance.

● ● ● DID YOU KNOW?

> Treatments normally last around 30 minutes, and around 15 to 20 treatments are usually recommended. This technique does not offer a permanent solution and should be combined with a good diet and exercise, but after the initial treatments, just one or two maintenance treatments a month may be sufficient.

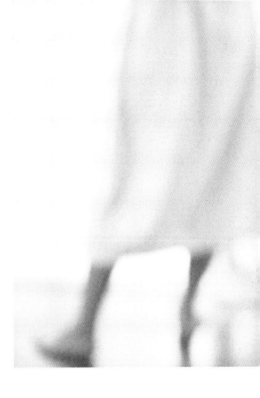

Deep massage

The patient generally wears an elasticated body stocking while a hand-held massaging device with adjustable rollers is passed over the affected areas, alternately sucking and rolling. The massaging action gently pinches the skin with controlled movements. This action has various benefits: it promotes the elimination of toxins and excess fluid, and also exfoliates. It has the effect of stimulating blood and lymphatic flow so that cellular function is improved.

The sensation is not unpleasant (it should not be painful) and can be quite relaxing, rather like a deep massage. A trained technician should be able to assess the level of massage that is suitable for you.

> As with many other treatments, body-rolling massage sessions are generally not cheap. Consult the Internet to find out what kind of treatments are on offer near you.

KEY FACTS

* Ensure you only use a trained and qualified practitioner at a respected spa or salon.

* The French, in particular, are at the forefront in the fight against cellulite and have developed many of the treatments currently on offer.

36

get rid of flabby thighs

Many women feel that they have flabby thighs. Exercises that mobilize the lower body are the best ways to tackle this problem. The following exercises are a good place to start the battle to tone your legs.

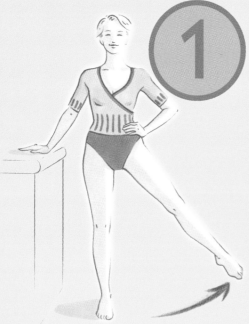

Exercise 1

Stand up straight next to a table, put one hand on the edge, the other on your waist. Bring the outside leg out sideways, with your toes pointing towards the ground. Raise your leg 20cm (9in) to the side. Hold the position, then bring your leg down again slowly. Breathe in and out deeply. Repeat the exercise ten times, then change sides. During the whole exercise, make sure that you don't move your pelvis, and keep you heel facing inwards.

Exercise 2

Get down on all fours, leaning on your left forearm. Slowly lift your right leg up to hip level, keeping your back perfectly straight. Lower it gently, without resting your knee on the floor. Repeat this ten times. Rest for a few moments, breathing deeply, then repeat the exercise with the left leg. Don't forget to do some stretching before and after your exercise. (See also Tip 26.)

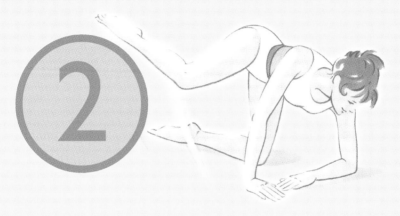

> Morning and evening, massage localized areas, either with your hands (working in a clockwise direction) or with a roller (see Tip 30). Finish off with a slimming cream.

> If your flabby thighs resist all your efforts, you could consider liposuction (see Tip 39).

> If you also have cellulite on your knees and inner thighs, the same operation may solve several problems at once.

KEY FACTS

* Precede all exercises with some breathing and stretching, with the window open.

* Cycling is also an excellent means of avoiding or reducing unwelcome extra weight on the hips.

37 firm your skin

Loss of elasticity of the skin often goes hand in hand with cellulite. There can be no anti-cellulite treatment without a complementary treatment to firm the skin.

Problem skin Researchers in the United States have put forward the theory that cellulite is less of a weight problem and more of a skin problem. Fight this curse by firming up the skin in order to resist the invasion of fat cells. But just how do you firm flesh that, thanks to a sedentary life and lack of treatment, tends to

wobble? Firstly, by boosting circulation. Exfoliate the skin with a scrub cream, shower, massage. Anything that stimulates and reddens the skin (although nothing too aggressive) is good for it.

The treatments After exfoliating apply a firming cream. Among the most effective are products containing vegetable and marine extracts enriched with a fortifying combination of ingredients, such as *Centella asiatica* and milk proteins. Also very efficient is a D-panthenol formula, sesame oil and lactic acid. There are many new products on the market that claim to firm your skin.

●●● DID YOU KNOW? ─────

> Plants, vegetable extracts (soya, grape) and marine extracts are commonly included in the formulas of firming treatments.
> Some include anti-free radical elements (vitamin E, green tea, sesame). All these should be rapidly absorbed and cause no discomfort.

KEY FACTS

* Remodelling creams that firm and tone your skin are one way to tackle cellulite.

* But these treatments do not mean you should give up sport.

38 tone your thighs

When the inside of your thighs becomes distended and the skin wrinkles, your morale falls. So do something about it by getting active.

First, tone your adductor muscles Jogging, cycling, swimming, dancing, horse-riding and skiing can all contribute to your 'perfect thighs' programme. If these activities are not available to you, look for a nearby gym or exercise studio where you can reap similar rewards.

Quick exercise, slim thighs Lie down on your side. With your head resting on your hand, bend the top leg and place your heel in front of the knee of the other leg, then lift this leg. Hold the position for two seconds. Relax, then repeat five times. Breathe deeply, then change sides.

Lie on your back, arms down by your side. Bend your legs and lift them 10cm (4in) off the floor. Tensing your abdominal muscles, move your heels apart and then back together. After ten repeats, rest. Then do another ten repeats.

KEY FACTS

* For these exercises to be efficient, make sure you do them slowly every day.

* You can do stretching exercises at any age (they improve balance and joint condition) and are suitable for everyone.

39 liposuction: the ultimate solution

Twenty-five years after its invention, liposuction is now one of the most common plastic-surgery operations. For many women with localized cellulite, it is *the* solution.

> Severely affected knees respond especially well to liposuction. Within a month, you could be wearing that miniskirt that has hung untouched in the closet for years.

● ● ● DID YOU KNOW?

> The liposuction technique was perfected in France in 1977 by Dr Jacques Illouz.

Definitive and effective

Liposuction is the only technique that provides a definitive solution for both widespread and localized cellulite (thighs, stomach, spare tyre). However, if you abandon your balanced diet, the fat will reform. The operation restores the skin's muscle tone and has a curative action on the circulation (blood vessels are no longer congested with cellulitic nodules). What's more, the psychological uplift it brings gives you a youthful bloom, whatever your age. (See also Tip 33.)

Find a good practitioner

This technique was previously reserved for deep fat (flabby thighs). Nowadays, though, the use of extra-fine tubes and the great skill of the specialists make it possible to treat superficial cellulite without leaving marks. Nevertheless, it's important to remember that this is a surgical procedure and it must be performed properly: the choice of surgeon is vital. Be aware that, if the procedure is not successful, it could result in complications such as lumpy-looking skin, scarring, numbness, swelling or even more serious, life-threatening conditions. Make sure you discuss the operation and its likely outcome in advance with your doctor and surgeon. It's not a cheap option, but if you really can't stand your stomach or thighs any more, and if you've tried innumerable courses of anti-cellulite creams and gels and have never seen good results, it could turn out to be money well spent in the long run.

KEY FACTS

* The operation is preceded by a consultation with the surgeon and some tests.

* Exposure to the sun after the operation is not recommended.

* Plan for a week of rest at home after the procedure.

> For your peace of mind before undertaking what is, after all, a surgical operation, avoid any plastic surgeon who advertises in the back pages of magazines. Get a list of respected, well-qualified, experienced practitioners from your local health authority.

40 visit a marine spa

Thalassotherapy is all about pure pleasure. You will be thoroughly pampered, see your cellulite attacked, and will return home bursting with knowledge about diets and lifestyle changes that you can implement on a day-to-day basis.

The benefits of sea water The chemical composition of sea water is close to that of human plasma. Rich in minerals and trace elements that can easily penetrate the skin, it has an invigorating effect on the body. The majority of spas offer anti-cellulite and slimming treatments, as well as impedancemetry (see Tip 42), hyper-protein slimming table, dietetics courses, affusions, wraps, massages, lymphatic drainage, gym and aqua-aerobics.

'Thalassa', the Greek for sea Thalasso-therapy offers all the benefits of the sea on dry land. It makes use of seawater and its by-products (mud, seaweed) to balance the skin's pH, exfoliate, hydrate and detoxify. Energy levels soar and you leave feeling radiant and full of good resolutions to take control of your life and maintain a healthy regime. Many women return for treatment year after year.

● ● ● DID YOU KNOW?

> The pressure that sea water exerts on your body is also good for vein and lymphatic problems.
> Thalassotherapy treatments are good for blood circulation problems, excess weight and stress, as well as other medical conditions.
> The centres, not unnaturally, are normally located by the coast.

KEY FACTS

∗ At certain times of the year spas have all-inclusive offers (treatment and accommodation) that cut their prices significantly.

∗ Due to its density, sea water lightens the body, giving you a workout without exerting yourself.

case study

I accepted there were some things I couldn't have, and now I'm happy looking at my bathroom scales

« A hyperactive rhythm, stress, meals on the run followed by a few big blowouts, and I found I'd put on 4kg (9lb). With that extra weight on my figure, and cellulite dimpling on my thighs, I looked ten years older. I was getting breathless running for the bus or going up four flights of stairs. I went to see my doctor. The blood tests came back with bad results: cholesterol, high sugar! He sent me to a dietician, and together we formulated a diet: not a starvation diet, but a reasonable one. Among the forbidden foods were butter (I love savouries!), sauces, ready-meals and, of course, those chocolate cakes! At first it was very hard, but after one month I had lost almost 2kg (4½lb). The weight loss slowed after that, but it was still coming off, and I felt so much better in myself. In six months, I'd lost the 4kg I'd gained, and I'm no longer afraid of the scales. I can fit in my old clothes again, and my orange-peel skin has gone too, with the help of the beauty parlour. Thank you, Doctor! »

41 »»»

» **Hard to the touch, often painful when pinched,** it affects various areas: hips, knees, buttocks, the inner thighs and, after fifty, even the upper arms.

»» Irrespective of whether it is accompanied by loss of elasticity of the skin (which is common), **established cellulite needs pro-active care and in-depth treatment**.

»»» In addition to sport and a balanced diet, it is often necessary to seek help from an aesthetic surgeon, and maybe even resort to plastic surgery. If you have reached this stage, you have two options: **either do something about it or accept that you will be able to wear only baggy clothes.** The choice is yours.

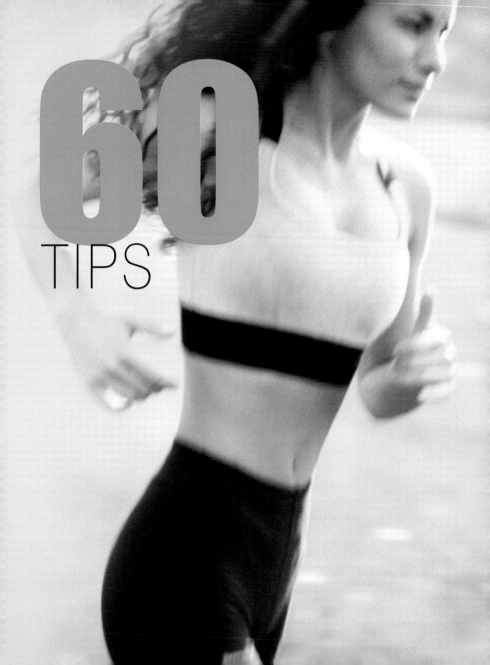

60
TIPS

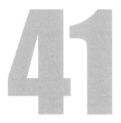

41

the root
cause

Why do you have a proliferation of fat cells? A biological disorder, inactivity, sheer greed, overwork, depression? Ask your doctor, then seek help from a specialist who will help you address your problem.

The dietary coach

Who needs a coach? More often than not, those who have dieted yo-yo-style and no longer know where to start to lose weight. The first aim must be to stop gaining any more. 'We don't propose anything revolutionary,' explains Patricia Juan of the Du Vernet Centre, 'just eating differently, building muscle, dislodging

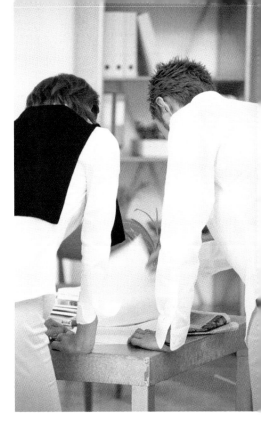

fat cells.' Every week, sample menus are drawn up and the previous week's lapses measured. After several carefully supervised consultations you will be back on the right track and given genuine encouragement to achieve your goal.

The therapist: unblocking blockages

When you can't bring wayward eating habits under control or are undergoing a period of depression, going to see a psychotherapist is a good way of helping you to see a light at the end of the tunnel. The root causes of your problems will be investigated and then treated accordingly, whether in behavioural therapy (private or group) or with a psychologist whose role is to research the psychological origins of your eating problems. Some plastic surgeons arrange a consultation for their patients before operating in the knowledge that stability of mind will give the surgery and recovery a much greater chance of success.

KEY FACTS

* Getting help is not a sign of weakness.

* In the case of significant excess weight, a doctor can prescribe a specialized thermal spa with psychotherapy.

42 update your scales

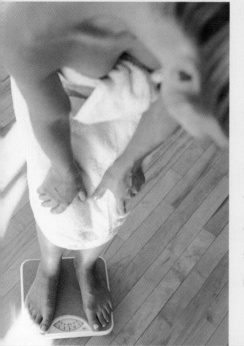

Getting on the scales every morning to keep track of every gram or ounce lost is pointless. Even if you do appear to have lost weight, it may simply be water rather than fat. But there is now an alternative to traditional bathroom scales that enables you to know exactly how you are progressing.

Do scales tell the whole story?

We now know that weighing yourself once a week is sufficient. Weighing yourself every day is meaningless. Various factors (dietary lapses, stress, intestinal transit, menstrual cycle) cause variations in your weight, and getting on your scales every morning won't make the fat disappear any faster. What's more, these days, we know that the weight shown isn't what really matters. With scales, you have no idea how much of your weight comprises fat and how much is muscular mass. But you can discover this through impedancemetry – a method of measuring the electrical resistance of the body. This is used in hospitals in the treatment of obesity, as well as in slimming treatment centres (thermal and marine spas, beauty parlours).

Impedancemetry and calories

Impedancemetry and precise electronic scales have become essential tools when dieting. As your weight is read, a small electric current is passed through the body (you feel nothing). Resistance is calculated in micro-amperes, the total weight analysed and the body fat index calculated. All of this is possible as lean mass contains more water and has a lower electrical resistance than fat, so the more fat you have, the higher your resistance to the electrical current. Some impedance meters also give the total number of calories to be consumed over 24 hours to remain at the indicated weight. Use this is a guideline, but don't let it become an obsession.

 KEY FACTS

* Weigh yourself at the same time of day (ideally at the end of the afternoon) and in the same conditions.

* Wait three to four hours after a meal before weighing yourself.

> Some impedance meters are designed for family use, including children from age seven upwards. They include a memory so you can see how you are progressing.

43

cook well and cook light

If you want to lose weight, you need to rethink the way you eat. Until now, perhaps you have been cooking without bothering too much about nutritional balance. Perhaps you need to change your ways.

Fundamental cooking methods

Dieticians say it repeatedly: steamed food is light and full of flavour. The steam passes through the food gently, ensuring optimal conservation of vitamins and minerals. It is a method that suits everything: meat, fish, vegetables, even fruit (a peach steamed in a foil parcel with a little cinnamon is delicious). Make light meals but, at around eleven in the morning, have a snack. Similarly, enjoy a cup of tea in the afternoon and you won't be tired or starving waiting for dinnertime. Forget pastries (sugar is transformed into fat) and snack on apples: with moderate sugar content (12 per cent), an apple contains vitamins and minerals, is filling and has a diuretic effect.

Don't punish yourself just for the sake of it

You don't have to deny yourself every culinary pleasure in order to lose weight. There's no point in restricting yourself to non-fat yoghurts if you hate them and love the 'full-fat' ones. 'Normal' yoghurt contains just 1g of lipids, which equates to a mere 9 calories more than skimmed-milk yoghurt. Or, to put it another way, it is the equivalent of two chips or a thin slice of sausage. Whether they are labelled 'low fat' or not, all yoghurts contain the same amounts of calcium and protein. Just avoid products that are high in sugar and have added flavouring.

> If you are craving chocolate, drink a glass of sparkling mineral water (it will fill you up). Take your mind off it, go out, browse in the local bookshop or go window shopping.

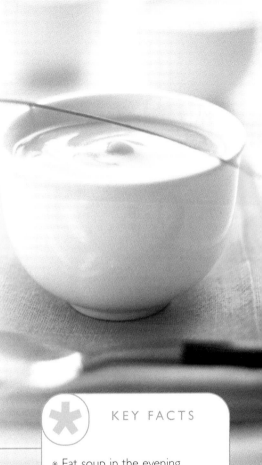

KEY FACTS

∗ Eat soup in the evening.

∗ Vitamin-rich slimming purée: 1 apple, half bunch of watercress, 5 sprigs of parsley, tarragon and mint. Purée and add a dash of single cream.

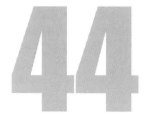

It's not rocket science: to shift your cellulite, you need to increase your physical activity significantly, and not only in the gym, but by incorporating endurance sports.

run, cycle, swim

Fat or muscle, the choice is yours

Nutritionists and slimming experts advocate physical exercise because they know that wherever you build muscle it will leave no room for fat. If you have calculated your BMI (see Tip 22), you will know your body mass index. If it is over 30, you need to rebalance your diet immediately. But to have the satisfaction of feeling slim and discovering a more toned body, you also need to take up a

> Slim down cellulitic knees and ankles by walking in the shallow end of the swimming pool with the water halfway up your calves. Start by doing 10 minutes, then working up to 15 for a real anti-cellulite massage.

> Finish off with a massage, applying an anti-cellulite cream. (See Tip 30.)

> Running in a group is motivational, but be careful to join one that is of a similar ability to yourself. There's nothing worse than being left behind by everyone else.

> Weak back? Before you buy gym equipment, seek your doctor's advice.

physical activity. Motivate yourself by repeating that fat takes up more space than muscle, so building muscle will make you slimmer.

Minimum of 40 minutes per session

Exercise doesn't have to mean going to the gym. Turn down lifts, don't use the car on short journeys and use the stairs rather than escalators or lifts. Ideally, alternate gym exercises and weight training (concentrate on your abdominal muscles) with an endurance sport, such as cycling, swimming or speed walking. Since you want to work on your whole figure, try to vary these activities. Working out in the gym and cycling trim the waist, build up your abdominal muscles and buttocks and shape your thighs and calves. The level of exertion should be progressive, but the objective, after two or three weeks of developing fitness and stamina, is to increase your energy expenditure. For it to pay off, a session should last between 30 and 45 minutes at an average intensity. Moderate exertion for an hour is more efficient than 20 minutes at a frenetic pace and several sessions a week are better than one mega-session once a week. Breathe deeply – oxygen 'eats' fat.

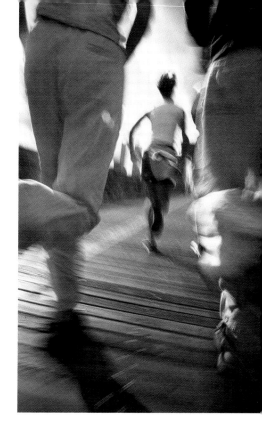

 KEY FACTS

* All exercise sessions should start and finish with stretching.

* If you are running, you must invest in proper shoes that are cushioned for shock absorption.

45

dip your toe into reflexology

For 5,000 years, Chinese medicine has been treating the whole body through the soles of the feet. Excess weight and cellulite are no exceptions: they can both be successfully treated via the reflex zones.

Genetics, stress, hormones, lifestyle

Feet are much more important than the Western world believes. Chinese medicine has identified 60 reflex points on the sole of the foot and produced an accurate map of them. There are also 7,000 nerve endings that correspond, via the spinal cord and the brain, to every part of the body. The principle of reflexology is that an imbalance of the body alters the magnetic field in the reflex

●●● DID YOU KNOW?

> Reflexology acts on fat, even when it is well established. It also has an impact on food cravings and venous efficiency.
> After a session, you might feel either tired or invigorated; both of these reactions are common and harmless.

> At the beginning, three to five sessions of 30 minutes to 1 hour may be needed, then one monthly session will normally suffice. The first session will include a preliminary talk with the practitioner.

zones. 'Excess weight', explains David Tran, a reflexologist, 'is the result of an energy imbalance. The reflex point that we stimulate depends on the causes, be they genetic, or due to stress, hormones or diet.'

Fat burning

Whatever the cause of the problem, the practitioner works on your inner energy, kneading and exerting pressure on various points on the sole of your foot, stimulating the organs concerned. If the excess weight is of dietary origin, he will give advice on how to amend your diet. Sometimes the results are rapid, with fat starting to disappear after two weeks although at other times the patient might not notice any improvement for a month.

> **Reflexology treats the whole person. It is suitable for stress-related conditions, sleep disorders, sports injuries and many other problems. It is not recommended for pregnant women. Consult your doctor if you have any concerns.**

KEY FACTS

* Still a mystery to many, reflexology is a good way to respond to the stresses of modern life.

* Irrespective of whether you are overweight, reflexology sessions will help you to relax and boost your energy levels.

46 feel good in your fifties

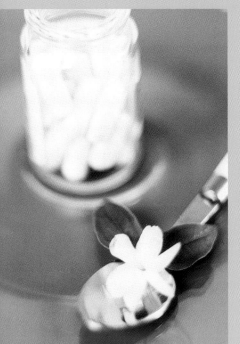

In your sixth decade, you will find that you gain weight more easily than ever before, and cellulite won't be far behind. After a check-up, the order of the day is often a new dietary regime. You can also try detoxing and/or protein products.

Sophisticated techniques make it possible to extract the best of the plant so that its active constituents can be used in creams and treatments.

Identify the problem

During the menopause, the secretion of oestrogen gradually ceases, which allows for the development of 'android' fat. It appears in new areas, creeping on to the buttocks, stomach, abdomen, arms, shoulders and breasts.

For a woman, turning fifty is a delicate time. Although it is a physiologically normal stage, you may not feel very good about yourself. Go and see your gynaecologist for a check-up, talk to him or her about whether you should have hormone replacement therapy. HRT has a favourable impact on fatty tissue and replaces some of the natural substances produced in a woman's body, but it is a complicated treatment and you should take advice from your doctor.

Diet and detox with care

With age, the elimination process becomes less efficient. Water is retained in the tissues and there is a natural tendency to gain weight, but lose height. The body needs a tailored response. There are food supplements to aid the elimination of toxins designed for women in their fifties. Ask your pharmacist for a natural product containing vegetable extracts selected for their cleansing qualities (yam, rosemary, olive tree, chicory, celery seed). A one-month treatment should make you feel lighter. As far as your diet is concerned, remember that you are not a kid any more: weight gain will be centred on your lower body. A starvation diet will make you lose weight from the top half, which means you risk a sagging face and bust. It might be advisable to consult a doctor about liposuction in the areas where you have a problem.

KEY FACTS

* It's far more difficult to eradicate cellulite at fifty than it is at thirty.

* The jury is still out on whether HRT causes cancer, heart disease and strokes.

> In order to build muscle, the body needs a constant source of protein. Protein makes you feel full and helps avoid muscle wasting. In your fifties, soya protein may be recommended.

47

trust in
aqua-aerobics

Aqua-erobics is an excellent form of aerobic exercise. Walking and jogging underwater strengthens the leg and hip muscles. Performed in shallow water, it frees the body of weight and allows you to build muscle gently.

Work without effort

The good news is that in water we weigh next to nothing (a mere 20 per cent of our weight), so the stresses and strains on the body during exercise are greatly reduced. You will find that you can increase the intensity of your activity quickly without suffering from the muscle ache you might be expecting. So aqua-aerobics is perfect for improving your physical condition without damaging your body in the process. You will soon be working effortlessly with floats, rings and foam bars. Two sessions per week are ideal. Followed by a few lengths of the pool at a good pace, this will improve your general condition (particularly the blood circulation at knee level, muscle tone on the arms and shoulders, and back strength) and shape your body.

Legs, hip and buttock exercise

Stand in water up to your waist with your right foot flat on the bottom, your left leg slightly raised to the side, toes pointed and back straight. Hopping on your right leg, bring your left leg in front of the right, without moving your pelvis, breathing in (the left foot remains pointed). Still hopping, now bring the left leg behind the right one, tense your buttocks and breathe out. Repeat twenty times on each leg.

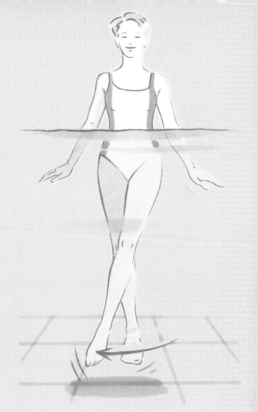

● ● ● DID YOU KNOW?

> For those who can't stand the smell of chlorine, some health clubs and spas use pine and cedar essences.

> Aqua-aerobics is a top treatment at thalassotherapy centres.

> Check out your local pool – most have aqua-aerobic sessions.

KEY FACTS

* Go regularly. If you can increase your aqua-aerobics sessions to three or four times a week, the results will be rapidly visible.

* After showering, treat yourself to a massage with a moisturizing slimming treatment.

48

take a look at mesotherapy

This technique stimulates blood circulation and eliminates toxins. Mesolift improves the appearance of cellulite and tones the skin; with mesolyse, you can reduce the width of your thighs by 2–5cm (1–2in).

Slim your thighs

Initially a medical treatment used in sports medicine and to relieve some pain (arthritis, migraine), mesotherapy particularly suits those who suffer from cellulite accompanied by circulatory problems. The doctor uses a mesotherapy gun to give you micro-injections of draining products, homeopathic or caffeine formulas just below the surface of the skin. This results in more efficient blood circulation and the elimination of toxins, with a consequent visible improvement in cellulite. Mesotherapy is also offered as a beauty treatment to combat hair loss.

Complementing the treatment through your diet

There are two types of treatment: the mesolift (one needle) for improved circulation and the mesolyse (several needles) that slims the thighs. Doctors who practise these techniques generally emphasize from the very first treatment that to obtain good results you must also reduce your fat and sugar intake. It's worth the effort. If you are sensible, the width of your thighs can be significantly reduced, and you'll lose the dimpling on your skin.

> Ensure that your mesotherapy practitioner always uses disposable needles. Do not undergo mesotherapy if you are likely to have an allergic reaction to any of the substances used. Consult a practitioner to be sure.

KEY FACTS

* The injections sting a little but any pain experienced is generally only minor and short-lived.

* For mesotherapy to be effective, you must also balance your diet: reduce your intake of fat and sugar (see Tip 49).

It can't be said often enough: eating fats and sugars will make your cellulite flourish. So you need to limit your consumption. Help yourself to resist them by discovering why you like them so much.

49

control lipids and carbohydrates

Lipids, brakes on your digestion

The human body cannot live without fat: it provides energy and is vital for cell formation. Every cell in your body is wrapped in a fine film of lipids: the cellular membrane. Packed with energy, fat is twice as calorific as carbohydrate or protein. It is also essential for the transportation of certain vitamins (E, A and D) that possess anti-ageing properties. Furthermore, lipids are good hunger regulators: fat takes a long time to digest,

●●● DID YOU KNOW?

> Cereals and potatoes themselves don't make you fat; the deep frying and rich dressings cause the damage.
> Eating bread, pasta, rice and potatoes will force you to reduce consumption of simple sugars and fat (you won't have the room), which improves your dietary balance.
> Of 100g (4oz) of carbohydrate consumed, 60g (2½oz) are stored in the liver (for energy); 25g (1oz) are used by the brain, kidneys and red blood

which means you feel full for longer and your blood-sugar level remains stable. That's why a pork chop covered in a rich, creamy sauce fills you up more than a steamed fillet of sole. How can you off-set it? Team it with pasta, for example, which contains slow sugars that will give you a lasting feeling of fullness.

Carbohydrates: sweetness rediscovered

Carbohydrate is the scientific term for various kinds of sugar: simple sugars (saccharose, fructose and glucose, which are present in sugar itself and sweet foodstuffs such as candy, jams, honey and fruit); complex sugars (starches, found in rice, bread, pasta, potatoes and legumi-nous vegetables); and non-digestible carbohydrates (found in fruit, vegetable and cereal fibre). Simple sugars are supremely tempting, but the body is supremely efficient at turning them into

fat (a moment on the lips, a lifetime on the hips). You will find it easier to resist them by increasing your consumption of complex sugars: they promote the secretion of serotonin, the good-mood hormone, so you still get pleasure from eating them, but they don't present the same hazards to your figure.

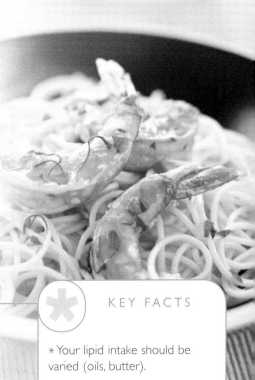

cells; and 15g (¹/₂oz) go to the muscles for their immediate needs and are partially transformed into fat as an energy reserve. Every gram you don't burn could be deposited somewhere on your figure.

50 do a DIY massage

Massaging your cellulite-dimpled skin pays off. You can do this on dry skin, or, if you are in a hurry, in the shower. Apply a cream afterwards.

Slim through massage Massage has long been known to aid localized slimming. It improves micro-circulation, boosts cellular exchange and prepares the skin for the application of slimming products. You can find massage shaping-stimulators at your pharmacy, comprising a glove and soap. The short, rounded knobbles on the glove allow a pressure-suction movement; the openings allow the penetration of an active mousse with decongesting plant extracts. Women with delicate skin can find tulle puffs on the beauty product shelves, which foam the soap and perform gentle exfoliation. Any moisturizing cream should then be absorbed easily.

Treatment products After the massage, use medicated treatment products sold in gel form at your pharmacy. They are the result of extensive laboratory research. A caffeine-based product contains an anti-drying ingredient that promotes its absorption deep-down in the cellulitic mass. Anti-fat, it decongests and activates local micro-circulation.

● ● ● D I D   Y O U   K N O W ?

> Help your varicose veins by putting up your feet when resting.
> Sit down with your legs stretched out in front of you and massage in an upwards direction using light, circular movements.

K E Y   F A C T S

✳ Dry your skin carefully and avoid rubbing.

✳ Finish off by apply a slimming moisturizing cream.

51 don't give up

When results remain elusive, despite all your efforts, will-power inevitably tends to flag. Avoid giving up and form a new plan of attack.

Expecting miracles? After three weeks of sensible eating and physical exercise, you feel lighter and fitter. But you have lost only 20 per cent of the weight you wanted to shed, and, despite the conscientious application of firming creams, your cellulite remains visible. You had hoped for so much more. Were you fooling yourself?

Stick with it Cellulite that has built up over months or years is difficult to shift. You can't get rid of excess weight and established cellulite in just a few weeks. If you are starting to despair, take a long, hard look at what you have been doing up to now. Perhaps it's time to choose a more aggressive approach: get a personal trainer; see a psychologist; invest in a course at a health spa. Get together with a group of like-minded friends and meet regularly to encourage each other and to boost your morale.

KEY FACTS

* Winter marine spas abroad allow you to slim while you tan.

* Don't hate yourself because your friends seem to have shed more weight than you. It's simply counter-productive.

52

put your money on new techniques

Health spas and beauty salons have built up quite an armoury of anti-cellulite techniques and equipment. The choice can be quite bewildering. You may well have to save up for the treatment, but your adipocytes will be terrified!

Anti-cellulite weapons

If you want to attack established cellulite, you need to drain excess fat from the adipocytes or remove them with surgery. If you cringe at the thought of the knife, place your trust in new techniques. Various machines are now available to combat all degrees of cellulite in all parts of the body. (See Tip 35.)

● ● ● DID YOU KNOW?

> The objective of these techniques is to tone and shape the figure, but they should not be used in isolation. In addition to any special treatments, it is important to follow a sensible, balanced diet and to take plenty of exercise. However, many of the techniques are not suitable for pregnant women. If you know or suspect you may be pregnant, always inform the doctor or technician before embarking on any course of treatment.

> Make sure you drink enough water to assist the detoxifying process.

Ultrasound, state of the art

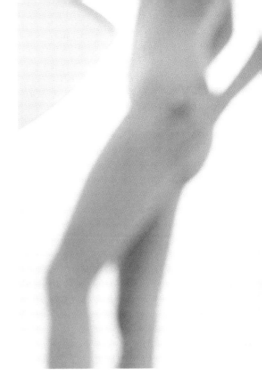

Some treatments are used in conjunction with others. Ultrasound is one such treatment, sometimes used in conjunction with liposuction (see Tip 39). This is another treatment that has been 'borrowed' from the area of medicine. It uses the same technology as that used to make ante-natal scans of pregnant women; only in the case of cellulite, the ultrasound waves penetrate just a few millimetres beneath the surface of the skin, affecting the adipose tissue where the cellulite is lodged. The ultrasound waves work by causing the cells in the body's tissue to vibrate. As they do so, fatty deposits are broken down, stimulating the elimination of toxins and waste products.

A typical session may begin with some bodybrushing and the application of special skin products designed to exfoliate and stimulate micro-circulation, prior to the ultrasound. There may be a session of massage after the ultrasound treatment, to promote the drainage of toxins via the lymphatic system.

KEY FACTS

* Ultrasound is non-invasive, but it is not cheap. Make sure you get the most out of your session (and your financial investment) by deciding to make some lifestyle changes and sticking to them.

* Laboratories are constantly striving to come up with new treatments. Keep an eye on the press for the latest treatments.

53

build up your abs
but mind your back

Slack abdominal muscles give you a flabby tummy.
You might even find cellulite developing there, too.
Build up your muscles and the fat will disappear.
Carefully designed exercises are essential if you
don't want to end up with a bad back.

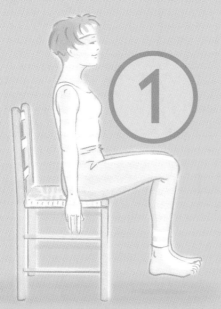

Two gentle movements

❶ Sitting on the edge of a chair, back straight, leaning slightly forwards, bring your knees together while parting your feet. Rest for about 20 seconds and repeat at least 10 times.

❷ Stand against a wall, chin tucked in, feet 30–45cm (12–18in) apart with your heels around 20cm (8in) from the wall. Pull in your stomach, clench your buttocks and tense the muscles of your perineum. Repeat 10 times.

The safe way to a sculpted stomach

You can buy excellent equipment that will help you build up your abdominal muscles safely in sports shops and by mail order. One such piece of equipment, the ab-trainer, is a metal frame that supports you correctly while enabling you to lift the upper part of your body without risking damage to your neck or back. Use it for a few minutes each day and you will develop the muscles necessary for a sculpted tummy. Ab-trainers routinely come with a videotape and booklet to guide you through the exercises step by step.

.

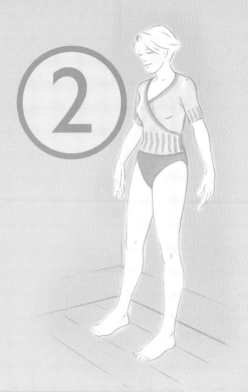

● ● ● DID YOU KNOW?

> It is important to work your upper and lower abdominals and your side abdominals, which shape the waist.

> All exercises should be done slowly, without straining. If you feel pain, stop; if the pain persists, see your doctor.

> Make sure you breathe in and out slowly.

KEY FACTS

* Ten minutes every morning will take ten years off you.

* Good abdominal muscles improve your posture.

54 sign up for stretching

Stretching courses are increasingly popular. They offer a gentle way to improve flexibility, while aiding relaxation and generating a welcome feeling of well-being.

Stretch out and relax Modern life is sometimes at odds with our bodies' needs. Stretching gently allows you to develop postures that will, among other benefits, boost your blood and lymph circulation, tone your muscles and slim your figure. Ideally, choose a course that takes place in the late afternoon, which is a good time for relaxation. Ensure that the session occurs in a pleasant atmosphere, then let the stretches do the rest. Half an hour should be enough to enable you to relax totally.

Supple and serene Combine gentle stretches with slow breathing; some stretching exercises relax a knotted back, while others generate energy or restore suppleness. When carried out properly, stretching can do more than just improve flexibility and ease muscular tension. It also leads to improved fitness, reduces the severity of painful periods and reduces the risk of injury to muscles and tendons during sporting activity.

● ● ● DID YOU KNOW?

> Stretching realigns the body and enhances the development of body awareness. It also improves co-ordination.
> If possible, practise some stretching exercises several times a day.

KEY FACTS

✳ Stretching is a method that promotes a good feeling, in body and mind.

✳ All the positions should be accompanied by deep breathing.

55 pour on the sauce

Reducing your fat intake means cutting out butter and those ladlefuls of oil and mayonnaise. Make sure you don't lose out on flavour by introducing some spicy condiments and sauces into your cooking.

Check out your kitchen cupboards

Steamed fish can get boring, so you need to enhance flavours during cooking with a choice of condiments. Think about herbs: parsley, chervil, chives, tarragon and basil. Try some of the many types of mustard. If there are no capers, gherkins or pickles in your cupboards, buy some and use them, along with gourmet vinegars (sherry, balsamic, raspberry). Multicoloured peppercorns, paprika and cayenne pepper are all fabulous, natural flavour-enhancers. The more you use them, the less salt you will want, which is good for that spare tyre.

Featherweight sauce: tomato fondue

Remove the cores of two tomatoes, skin and deseed. Chop the flesh. Add the mashed-up yolk of a hard-boiled egg, a chopped stick of celery and a little olive oil. Add pepper to taste and mix.

● ● ● DID YOU KNOW?

> Add a pinch of curry powder to your rice.

> Single cream (or, better still, yoghurt), rather than double cream, can be used to make a sauce for steamed apples. Boost the flavour with a sprinkling of nutmeg.

> Fennel gives a delicious aniseed flavour to salads.

KEY FACTS

∗ Low-fat vinaigrettes contain three times less fat than normal versions.

∗ Take a look at flavoured semolina for a good alternative to high-fat desserts.

56

separate fact from fiction

You hear so many contradictory stories where slimming is concerned. Each new theory seems to say the exact opposite of the previous one. So, where exactly does the truth lie in the jungle of information now available to us on diet and lifestyle?

Diet

• 'Skipping breakfast makes you fat'. TRUE. You'll be so hungry that you'll probably crack and eat something sweet during the morning.
• 'A low-calorie drink won't help your cellulite'.
FALSE. It will satisfy your sugar craving and in doing so help prevent you gaining too much weight.

●●● DID YOU KNOW?

> A diet rich in nourishment and low in calories will help you to lose weight.

> Chew your food well and make sure your meals don't last less than 20 minutes. Otherwise, no matter what you are eating, you may have the sensation that you have not had quite enough.

> Power walking and jogging will get your circulation going as well as tone your legs and buttocks.

> Cycling is good low-impact exercise. It strengthens the muscles in the legs and helps to slim the knees and ankles.

- 'Eating at the same time every day is a good thing'.
TRUE. You are less likely to snack. Also, if the body never knows when it's going to eat next, it goes into storage mode.
- 'Meal substitutes and powdered protein are the same thing'.
FALSE. Meal substitutes do not contain protein.
'Eating sweets puts you in a good mood'.
TRUE. Sugars trigger the secretion of serotonin, the body's happy hormone.

Physical activity

- 'Working out at the gym makes you look fatter, even if you're not'.
FALSE. A kilo of muscle occupies less space than a kilo of fat.
- 'Having a sauna can't really help your cellulite'.
TRUE. It makes you sweat and you eliminate toxins and water, but it has no significant impact on accumulated fat.
- 'Lifting weights is the only thing that will get rid of fat on your arms'.
FALSE. Stretching is excellent and you won't risk inflammation of the joints.
- 'Around 8 litres (14 pints) of air per minute passes through the lungs of a person with a sedentary lifestyle. Sports people use much more'.
TRUE. People who play sports use almost double.

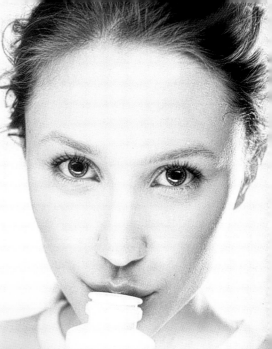

- 'Running doesn't have any effect on the brain'.
FALSE. When you exert yourself, the brain secretes endorphins, molecules that induce euphoria and relaxation.

 KEY FACTS

* Sport significantly helps reinforce the efficiency of your diet .

* It doesn't make you lose weight, but it tones the tissues and trims your figure.

57 consider slimming aids

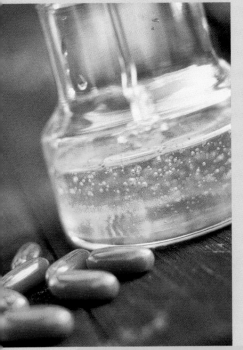

Investigate plant-based slimming supplements at your local pharmacy. Since you normally take them with a glass of water, they encourage you to drink more water too. The supplements help to eliminate toxins, curb the appetite and reduce fat absorption. All very useful slimming aids.

DID YOU KNOW?

> You will have seen it on every single packet, but it bears repeating: 'These special formulas can aid weight loss only as part of a calorie-controlled diet.'

> Slimming products are for internal use and cannot be given to children. Keep them out of reach of the very young: sugar-coated pills in brightly coloured boxes can look like sweets.

Detox and water retention

Look for supplements that aim to stimulate blood and lymph micro-circulation, eliminating toxins, waste and water trapped in the tissues. There are many different supplements on the market, and many contain plant extracts. Favourite among these are whole grape extract, green tea, and pineapple, and diuretic and depurative plants such as orthosiphon, meadowsweet, burdock, pilosella, briar, fennel, ash and dandelion. Algae is also used. It contains fibres that absorb water as food is being digested. Fruit-flavoured solutions and juices (such as pineapple) can also aid detoxing. An added bonus is that their pleasant tastes encourage you to drink more during the day.

Fight cravings

How can you diminish these cravings? Dietary supplements can help. For example, lupin and konjac induce calmness and a feeling of fullness and garnicia subdues sugar cravings. Apple pectin suppresses appetite, making you feel full for longer, so helping you lose weight.

> However much you want to lose weight, food supplements should be taken only for a limited period of time.

New appetite-suppressants are appearing on the market all the time.

Fat-burners

These products are intended for internal use and help eliminate fats that the body stores up. Among the more recent is a product made with guarana and *Citrus aurentium*: rich in vitamins and minerals, it accelerates digestion and metabolism and promotes the burning of fat. When used with a gel, it firms the tissues. Another useful extract is *Camelia sinensis*, which also accelerates fat burning. Chitosan, a fibrous extract from the skeletons of shellfish, can absorb up to 12 times its own volume. Fat in the stomach becomes attached to it before it can be absorbed into the digestive tract. It is then eliminated from the body.

KEY FACTS

* Don't try to combine several products. Their slimming potential will not be increased.

* Always read the instructions carefully if using a slimming aid, and make sure you drink at least the recommended amount of water when taking them.

58

take care of your knees

Are you ashamed of your knees? Have they become thick and puffy, sentencing you to a lifetime in trousers and long skirts? The trick is to get moving. Do some exercise, massage them and attack the cellulite that is spoiling them.

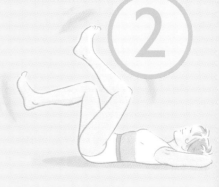

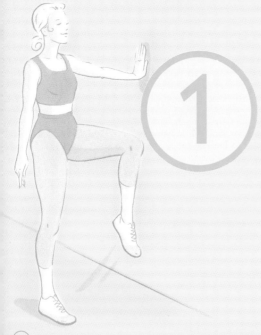

Stairs and flexing

Climb the stairs with a straight back and stretch each leg well on every step. Climbing stairs works the muscles and joints, strengthening the legs, so take the the stairs instead of the lift whenever you can. If you drop something, don't bend from the waist to pick it up; this stresses the vertebrae. Instead, keeping your back straight and, pulling in your abdominal muscles, bend your knees and slowly bend down to the floor. Then slowly come back up, relaxing your stomach. This is another simple exercise that you can do at any time during the day.

Three exercises to slim your knees

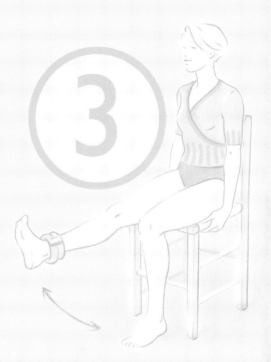

❶ Wearing flat shoes, stand with your left hand flat against a wall, bend your right leg and lift it in front of you, breathing in. Repeat 12 times, then do the same for the left leg.

❷ Lying down, hands behind your head, back flat against the floor, lift your legs and pedal towards the floor while breathing out and pulling in your tummy. Do three series of 10.

❸ Sit on a chair with your back flat against the chair back and your hands holding the arms, wearing a 500g (1lb) ankle weight. Lift your leg to the horizontal, then bend the knee in a fairly sustained rhythm while breathing gently out. Do three series of 20 flexes per leg, 3 times per week.

● ● ● DID YOU KNOW?

> Cycling and exercises carried out in the water tone the knees without being too tiring. Walk for 10 minutes in the swimming pool or the sea, with the water up to your mid-calves. This is good resistance exercise.

> If your knees are very swollen, you may wish to consider liposuction. (See Tip 39.)

KEY FACTS

✳ After exercise, massage your knees with a moisturizing slimming cream.

✳ Cycling reduces cellulite dimpling on the knees.

59

zap the cellulite at a thermal spa

Thermal spas all over the world now offer a wide range of new treatments, in addition to the more traditional ones. Increasing numbers of them now offer anti-cellulite treatments too.

Water and much more besides

Mineral water has been used to combat weight problems for over a century. But some thermal spas have recently moved up a gear in their slimming treatments. You can now benefit not only from the specific action of the thermal waters but from an arsenal of modern treatments, slimming massages, dietary information

● ● ● DID YOU KNOW?

> Thermal spas are not locked in the past. They have moved with the times and offer ultra modern facilities. The accommodation is often of a very high (and therefore expensive) standard.

> If staying in a spa hotel is too expensive, you could try renting a studio nearby and go in on a daily basis, just for the treatments.

and so on. You may also be able to indulge yourself in essential-oil baths, work out in aqua-aerobics and treat your skin with wraps. All spas have their own chefs whose job it is to concoct light but delicious meals bursting with flavour. The objective is to lose several pounds and return home feeling toned and fit.

Innovative ideas

Spas are at the forefront of research into slimming techniques. One such spa is the Royat-Chamalières, in the heart of the Auvergne in France. There, the usual array of showers, massages, gym workouts and baths are complemented by subcutaneous injections of thermal gas, which is said to have a beneficial effect on venous and arterial micro-circulation. The skin puffs up in a spectacular way, but it's a completely safe procedure. In one week, you can lose 1.5cm ($\frac{1}{2}$in) from around each thigh. The results last for several months, and venous insufficiency is significantly improved. This treatment is given under medical supervision.

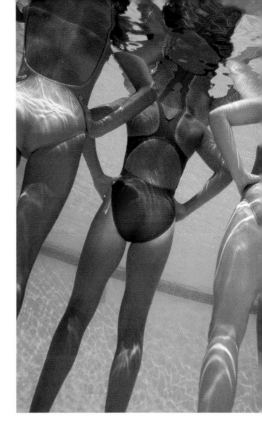

KEY FACTS

* The use of thermal waters (or hot springs) for therapeutic purposes dates back to Greek and Roman times.

* Spa treatments are not all frivolous fun. Some are performed under medical supervision.

60 treat yourself!

You've lost weight. Congratulations! You've shed a good deal of your cellulite, but some areas are still not perfect. You feel that you've got to be strict with yourself or you'll be right back where you began. But sometimes it pays to give in to temptation, just a little.

Be realistic Women often demand a lot of themselves, perhaps too much. You feel like giving up altogether. Don't! Be rational about it. You are not going to lose weight at 40 as easily as you did at 20. Just adjust your expectations.

Keep your sense of proportion A psychiatrist specializing in food behavioural problems, Dr Apfeldorfer, says: 'Many women approach slimming as if it were a battle, so if you want to succeed, you have to listen to yourself.' Be less exacting: from time to time, eat a little of something you really love. You are winning, so there's nothing wrong with letting your hair down a little every now and then.

KEY FACTS

* Every woman needs to find her own balance, and form.

* It's healthy to take pleasure in eating.

case study

My morale improved when I lost my tummy

« When you start wearing a blouse or a T-shirt over your skirt or trousers, it's because there's a problem: a little pot-belly. That's what I did, until I hit 45, after 3 pregnancies. Then I realized that it was making me look 10 years older. The aesthetic surgeon I consulted was clear about it: in my case, liposuction was the best and safest solution. It was going to cost a lot of money, but I could afford it if I didn't get the new car I'd had my eye on, didn't buy any new clothes and gave the hairdresser's a miss. At the end of the day, I figured it's better to look slim in a tatty pair of jeans than to bulge out of a piece of haute couture. I made an appointment with an aesthetic surgeon. The first interview convinced me and I felt confident from the start. Examination, photos, tests and then one morning I found myself on the table: general anaesthetic, two days in the clinic, a week at home, a girdle. Then, a perfect tummy. In six months, I will trust the same surgeon with my knees. We make a good team. »

useful addresses

» **Acupuncture**

British Acupuncture Council
63 Jeddo Road
London W12 9HQ
tel: 020 8735 0400
www.acupuncture.org.uk

**British Medical
Acupuncture Society**
12 Marbury House
Higher Whitley, Warrington
Cheshire WA4 4QW.
tel: 01925 730727

**Australian Acupuncture
and Chinese Medicine Assn**
PO Box 5142
West End, Queensland 4101
Australia
www.acupuncture.org.au

» **Jin shin do (*do-in*)**

www.jinshindo.org

» **Lymphatic drainage**

MLD^{UK} (professional association of manual lymphatic
drainage practitioners)
PO Box 14491, Glenrothes
Fife, Scotland KY6 3YE
tel: 01592 748008
www.mlduk.org.uk

» **Massage**

**British Massage Therapy
Council**
www.bmtc.co.uk

**Association of British
Massage Therapists**
42 Catharine Street
Cambridge CB1 3AW
tel: 01223 240 815

European Institute of Massage
42 Moreton Street
London SW1V 2PB
tel: 020 7931 9862

» **Plastic surgery**

**British Association of
Aesthetic Plastic Surgeons**
The Royal College of
Surgeons of England
35-43 Lincoln's Inn Fields
London WC2A 3PE
tel: 020 7405 2234
www.baaps.co.uk

**The Australian Society
of Plastic Surgeons**
Level 1, 33-35 Atchison St
St Leonards 2065
Sydney, Australia
tel: 1300 367446
www.plasticsurgery.org.au

**The American Society for
Aesthetic Plastic Surgery**
tel: 1 888 ASAPS 11 (toll-free)
www.surgery.org

» **Reflexology**

**The British Reflexology
Association**
Monks Orchard
Whitbourne
Worcester WR6 5RB
tel: 01886-821207
www.britreflex.co.uk

**Reflexology Association
of America**
4012 Rainbow Ste.
Las Vegas, NV 89103-2059
tel: 1-978-779-0255
www.reflexology-usa.org

**Reflexology Association
of Australia**
tel: 0500 502 250
www.reflexology.org.au

» **Yoga**

The British Wheel of Yoga
25 Jermyn Street
Sleaford
Lincs NG34 7RU
tel: 01529 306 851
www.bwy.org.uk

index

acknowledgements

Cover: R. Daly/Getty Images; p.8-9: H. Scheibe/Zefa; p.10-11: P. Curto/Getty Images; p.13: Miles/Zefa; p.14-15: P .Leonard/Zefa; p.17: B. Erlinger/Zefa; p.19: Ansgar/Zefa; p.20-21: Neo Vision/Photonica; p.24-25: B. Shearer/Option Photo; p.26-27: Neo Vision/Photonica; p.28: K. Reid/Getty Images; p.35: V. Besnault/Getty Images; p.38-39: Davies and Star/Getty Images; p.43: L. Adamski Peek/Getty Images; p.44: Neo Vision/Photonica; p.48-49: M. Kawana/Photonica; p.51: Emely/Zefa; p.53: Neo Vision/Photonica; p.54-55: Chabruken/Getty Images; p.57: B. Yee/Photonica; p.58: L. Beisch/Getty Images; p.62-63: E. Deshais/Marie Claire; p.65: I. Hatz/Zefa; p.67: S. Lancrenon/Marie Claire; p.70: S. Simpson/Getty Images; p.72-73: Star/Zefa; p.75: J. LeFortune/Zefa; p.77: J. Ieki/Photonica; p.82: Neo Vision/Photonica; p.86-87: P. Curto/Getty Images; p.89: Neo Vision/Photonica; p.90: J. Darell/Getty Images; p.92-93: Anthony-Masterson/Getty Images; p.95: E. Buis/Zefa; p.96-97: P. La Mastro/Getty Images; p.98: M. Montezin/Marie Claire; p.102-103: M. Rutz/Getty Images; p.104-105: L. Beisch/Photonica; p.109: B. Shearer/Option Photo; p.114-115: P. Baumann/Marie Claire; p.116: Miles/Zefa; p.121: D. O'Clair/Zefa.
Illustrations: Anne Cinquanta pages 22, 32-33, 40, 60-61, 78-79, 100-101, 110-111 and 118-119.

The author would like to thank the specialists who have assisted him: Dr J Boulet, homeopath; Dr Jean-Marie Bourre, nutritionist; Dr Alain Bzowski, aesthetic surgeon; Dr Michèle Freud, psychotherapist; Dr Michèle Lachowsky, gynaecologist; Dr Catherine Laverdet, dermatologist; Dr N Maguy, acupuncturist; Dr Jean Pierre de Mondenard, sports doctor; Dr Philippe Moinet, internist; M-F Six dietician; David Tran, reflexologist; Dr Jean-Philippe Zermati, nutritionist.

I would also like to thank the following laboratories, institutes and manufacturers: Centre Amak, Anne Sémonin, Arkopharma, Biotherm, Bleu comme Bleu, Caudalie, Dim, Christian Dior, Clarins, Darphin, Decléor, Elancyl, Esthederm, Galénic, Jeanne Gatineau, Guerlain, Guinot, Pierre Fabre, Juventhera, Estée Lauder, Lierac, Oenobiol, Orlane, Matis, Roc, Sisley, Spa Cinq Mondes, Thalgo, Vernet (Centre Du), Vichy, Yonka, Yves Rocher, Yves Saint Laurent, Centre Vareg, Centre Du Vernet.

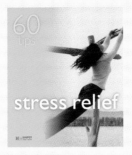
stress relief

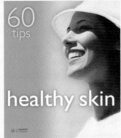
healthy skin

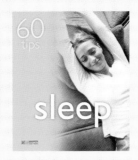
sleep

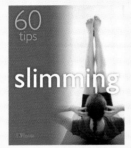
slimming

The 60 Tips collection All the keys, all the tips and all the answers to your health questions

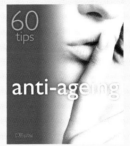
anti-ageing

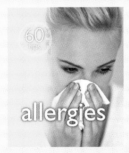
allergies

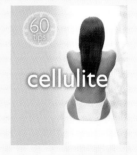
cellulite

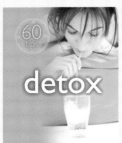
detox

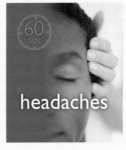
headaches

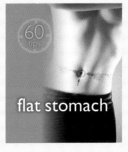
flat stomach

Series editor: Marie Borrel

Editorial director: Caroline Rolland

Editorial assistants: Caroline Rolland and Anne Vallet

Graphic design and layout: G & C MOI

Preparation, final checking: Maire-Claire Seewald and Fanny Morel

Illustrations: Guylaine Moi

Production: Felicity O'Connor

Translation: JMS Books LLP

© Hachette Livre (Hachette Pratique) 2003
This edition published in 2005 by Hachette Illustrated UK, Octopus Publishing Group Ltd.,
2–4 Heron Quays, London E14 4JP

English translation by JMS Books LLP (email: moseleystrachan@blueyonder.co.uk)
Translation © Octopus Publishing Group Ltd.

A CIP catalogue for this book is available from the British Library

ISBN-13: 978-1-84430-090-7

ISBN-10: 1-84430-090-0

Printed in Singapore by Tien Wah Press